SPELLBINDING

The Anglo-Saxon Runes,

Magic & The Soul

Kennan Taylor, MD

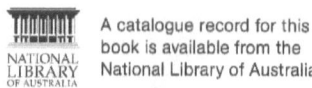
A catalogue record for this book is available from the National Library of Australia

Copyright © 2023 Kennan Taylor

Kennan Taylor asserts the moral right to be identified as the author of this work. Except as provided by Australian law, no part of this book may be reproduced without permission in writing from the author.

Contact details:
drkennan1@gmail.com

All rights reserved.
ISBN-13: 978-1-922727-76-3

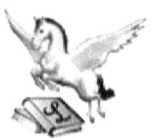

Linellen Press
265 Boomerang Road
Oldbury, Western Australia
www.linellenpress.com.au

Contents

Contents iii
Preface 1
Introduction 5
Introducing the Futhorc 12
The Anglo-Saxon Mentality 32
How to Use the Runes 40
    Introduction 41
    Getting to know the Runes 44
    Divination 45
    The Rune Journal 49
    Ritual 50
    Magic 52
    Rune Magic 53
The Anglo-Saxon Futhorc 57
    Introduction 57
    Addendum on Aetts: 64
    FEOH (F) - Wealth, Cattle 65
    UR (U) - Aurochs 68
    THORN (Th) - Giant, Thorn 71
    OS (O) - God, Mouth 74
    RAD (R) - Riding, Road 77

CEN (C) - Torch, Light 80
GYFU (G) - Gift 83
WYN or WYNN (W) - Joy, Pleasure 85
HAGAL or HAEGL (H) - Hail 88
NYD (N) - Need, Necessity 91
IS (I) - Ice 94
GER (Y) - Year, Harvest 97
EOH (EO) - Yew (tree) 100
PEORTH (P) - A Game 102
EOLH (X/Z) - Protection, Elk-sedge 104
TIR (T) - The God 109
BEORC (B) - Birch 112
EH (E) - Horse 114
MAN (M) - Man 116
LAGU (L) - Lake 118
ING (NG) - The God (or Frey) 120
ETHEL (OE) - Inherited Property 123
DAEG (D) - Day 125
The Rune Extension of the Futhorc 127
AC (A) - Oak 130
AESC (AE) - Ash 132
YR (Y) - Yew bow 134
IOR or IAR (EO or IO) - Fish, Eel or Serpent 136
EAR (EA) - Earth, soil 138
CWEORTH (Q) - Ritual fire 140
CALC (K) - Cup, Chalice 142

STAN (ST) - Stone	145
GAR (G) - Spear	147

Addenda 149
On Christianisation 149
Sexuality 150
Magic 151

Sample Readings 153
A Rune for the Day 154
A Divinatory Reading 155
Postscript 158
Medicine Wheel Reading 159

Postscript to the 33 Rune Futhorc 163
The Futhorc 163
Tradition 165
Other Disciplines 167

The Religious and Spiritual Context 169
Medicine 174
Magic 176
Sexuality 179

The Soul Complex 184
Introduction 184
The Old English Body-Soul Complex 189
Body-Mind 192
Beyond the Body-Mind 196
Reflections 201
The Body-Soul Complex in Modernity 204

The Personal Soul *205*
The Liminal Soul *207*
The Transpersonal Soul *209*
The Integrated Soul *211*
Conclusions and Relevance to the Runes *213*

Runes, Tarot, Alchemy & the Holy Grail **215**

Spellbinding **222**

Postscript **235**

Appendices **237**

The Anglo-Saxon Rune Poem **245**

The Norse Rune Poem **250**

The Icelandic Rune Poem **253**

Havamal **256**
Odin *256*

Bibliography **261**
General Runelore *261*
Anglo-Saxon Runes *261*

Biography **263**

Preface

This is not an academic work. It has no pretence to being unduly scholarly. It is a work to invite and draw you in to the magic of the runes, to see if they charm and enchant you. If they do, then there are pointers, both here and in the references, in how to explore this enchantment further; not just in theory, but also in practice.

The opinions expressed here are my own, born of inquiry and research. I do not pretend they are right in any absolute or objective sense, but they may provide a template for your experience and exploration to arrive at your own conclusions. Too often writers in these fields obscure their opinions behind so-called facts and research; a position I find to be disingenuous. Instead, this invitation is open-ended and you are free to party with or without me … or not party at all.

From the earlier more descriptive work, *Just Add Blood* that was more exclusively about the runes and how they could be used in a divinatory and basic magical manner, I have naturally explored and extended my interests further over time. I have drawn on other fields and disciplines, which I have explored in articles, papers and posts, where there has been a significant overlap with the whole field of runelore.

So, you may detect some emphases that deviate a fair way away from the subject of the runes, or even detect a different voice in the various sections. Rather than iron these out into some sort of uniformity and connect them together in a linear way, I have left the voices and meanderings largely unchanged and added links, where deemed necessary. So, unlike an ordered and planned work, this is more woven like a tapestry.

As I have moved from a basic to a more detailed integration of magic with my use of the runes, I have also found it necessary to understand the Anglo-Saxon or Old English mentality in more detail. This led to a lengthy detour into understanding the concept of the Soul, as experienced by peoples of the first millennium of our era, which is somewhat different from the way it is presented by the Church, particularly the Roman one. Whilst this exploration of the Soul leads into a relatively separate section of the book, it provides a perspective to look at magic, mysticism and healing that I have found very rewarding, but also relatively essential in understanding the runes and where they fitted into the culture of the time.

As a basic treatise on the runes and divination, this work now seems relatively complete, with avenues like bindrunes, magical usage and making one's own set in the hands of the reader. The inquiry into their magical usage is opened up; however, it is necessarily limited in a work such as this, although I think there is enough information provided – including in the bibliography – for those wanting to explore magical practice to proceed on their own.

The Soul inquiry is somewhat parallel to this, designed to get the reader into the mentality of the times and its inherent richness. Topics like spirituality, sex and even drugs, link the soul – as the centre and agent of life's journey – to pathways like the runes and their magical usage. Interwoven, like a tapestry, but open-ended and idiosyncratic, this book may be as valuable as the reader makes it.

This is a largely solitary work, written unaided and in a rather idiosyncratic and journalistic style. My work derives originally from medicine and psychotherapy; writing is a later creative addition to my professional armoury. I am still learning the ropes, including my written voice and style of presentation. The audience, I hope, is drawn from across the population at large, so I have tried to reach out to the niches in the various groupings who would be attracted to a work of this kind; generally, to those readers who have had enough theory and want more practical instruction.

More specifically, I would like to thank those within my own spiritual community, which consists of individuals in Western Australia that I serve in my capacity as Elder and Druid. The runes provide a magical backdrop not only to my healing practice, but to our work in ritual, ceremony, sweat house and feast.

I bless you all.

Introduction

SPELLBINDING is a personal study of the Anglo-Saxon or Old English runes and their usage and relationship to the Anglo-Saxon worldview, all written from a fundamentally psychospiritual perspective. It will serve both as a guide in *how to use the runes* and as an exploration into their significance, both traditional and contemporary, from a primarily magical perspective. Inevitably, this will have my own personal imprimatur in a vast, expanding, and often confusing field. The terms Anglo-Saxon and Old English are relatively synonymous, the latter being used more to reflect the development of the English language over time. I will refer to the more familiar and broader cultural term of *Anglo-Saxon* in this work, unless otherwise relevant, such as when discussing language.

The Anglo-Saxon runes are commonly referred to as the *Futhorc*. Named after the more familiar Roman letters that are used to identify the first six runes, the Anglo-Saxon Futhorc is the equivalent of the more familiar Germanic *Futhark* (often referred to as the *Elder Futhark*, to distinguish it from the shorter *Younger Futhark* that developed from the Elder Futhark in the later Viking era). The Elder Futhark is considered the prototypal rune set and has become popular in the modern era as a tool of divination, particularly in New Age circles. That this has led to a considerable amount of trivialisation is taken for granted, but this is not the reason I favour the Futhorc; it is because the Futhorc inclines not only to my own heritage (as well as that of many readers, as it is specifically Anglo-Saxon), but also because it captures spiritual concepts that I consider very relevant to our time and which are not included in the Germanic Futharks.

What I have decided to do, and differently from other works on the runes, is to add two significant sections on the Anglo-Saxon concept of the *Soul* (I will continue to capitalise the term Soul for emphasis, where and when I deem it appropriate), these being: the *Anglo-Saxon Mentality* and *The Soul Complex*. Initially, this was to provide a perspective of what might have been the mentality of the times, but then I wondered how the insights that I gained from this initially separate exploration would then inform and change my view of the Futhorc. These sections of the book are necessarily more idiosyncratic and speculative, but I hope they may help the reader in developing a sensibility not only in approaching the runes, but also providing insights onto their own spirituality and its direction.

This is not the only point of departure. I will be expanding on the concept of the Soul drawn from the religious understanding of it in the first millennium, linking it to some modern psychological and even medical views, and use it as a broader basis for appreciating modern spirituality more holistically. This will extend to an understanding of how runes, specifically the Futhorc, blended into religious and spiritual views, not only in the first millennium, but also extending through the mediaeval period to modernity. Christianity, and mystical concepts like the Grail, will be seen in a more integrated way than is commonly undertaken, so enhancing the story of the runes. Alchemy will be touched on as a major unifying theme in this regard and a short section devoted to its association to runes (specifically the Northumbrian extension), Tarot cards and the Grail in *Runes, Tarot, Alchemy & The Holy Grail*.

I will be bringing the body of knowledge around the runes, and the Futhorc in particular, into the world of magic. As this is not primarily an academic or research work; it promotes the idea that the runes are integral to a spiritual vision of life and our place in the universe. It also furthers our active involvement in this process, which is the domain of magic. But magic is not primarily a manipulation of material reality; it is understanding and working with the metaphysical forces that both underpin our physical existence and in which this existence is contained. I will be providing some insight into the magical arts, drawn from my study of the runes, which might make these arts more understandable, as well as approachable and useable in the modern everyday sense. These insights will be woven into relevant themes, such as sexuality throughout, the various interfacing with religion, and occasionally (as in the concluding *Spellbinding* section) to drugs and altered states of consciousness.

Finally, and maybe a little controversially, I will be elucidating in the *Spellbinding* section about how I am developing my own rune row, or rune set, to use personally and magically. What I am undertaking here is hardly sacrilege, it would have been how the runes and their variations developed in the first place, as acts of divine inspiration if you like. But it is also in the spirit of modernity; revitalising the forces contained in the runes and giving them a modern, as well as prophetic future expression.

A few words about the content and order referred to above, laid out in a more linear fashion:

- *Introducing the Futhorc* provides a more detailed context for the runes and to illuminate what has been called the Dark Ages, or Early Mediaeval period, being 400 – 1066 AD. Appreciation of this period gives a more grounded and traditional context for the runes, as well as relevance for and to the modern age.

- The *Anglo-Saxon Mentality* is outlined with reference to the concept of the *Soul*, as understood in this period. In contrast to our modern view, adopting this mentality – through the agency of the soul – provides a detailed understanding of the runes and their purpose.

- *How to use the Runes* may be ground the reader has already seen elsewhere, as it covers areas like ritual, divination and magic, as well as how to use a journal. However, it will give a perspective on how this book specifically approaches the Futhorc, so may be useful even to those experienced in these subjects.

- I then move into the *Anglo-Saxon Futhorc*, with various intentions. To provide continuity with the Germanic or Teutonic Traditions, but also to illustrate the differences between them, as well as the progression of Anglo-Saxon magic and spirituality within this period and beyond.

- *Sample Readings* is what it says: A practical outline of some straightforward ways of working with the Futhorc.

- The *Postscript* fills in any lingering gaps that may have emerged from the descriptions of the runes in the Futhorc and the discussion around them.

- *The Religious and Spiritual Context* then moves into the spiritual background to the Futhorc, past and present, and expands further on medicine, magic and sexuality within the context of this study.

- Now we move into *The Soul Complex*. This is a weighty area to cover, extending as it does from the *Anglo-Saxon Mentality*. It will be new ground for most, and is almost a "book within a book". As well as linking with modern scientific disciplines, it provides a deeper and richer background for what is to follow, but can be read in isolation or bypassed if straightforward *runelore* is what is desired.

- *Runes, Tarot, Alchemy & The Holy Grail* illustrates the broader context of the runes beyond their straightforward use in magic and divination. Although speculative, the Futhorc is specifically identified as containing alchemical themes and a relationship to the Tarot and spiritual legends, such as The Holy Grail.

- *Spellbinding* will examine the differences between the runic and Roman scripts in more detail. Then the concept of the bindrune – used elsewhere – will here focus on how to combine the runes for deeper significance, as well as to provide a basis for their magical usage.

- The *Appendices* provide the background and detail referred to, but not always included in the main text.

- A short *Bibliography* follows, as I have decided not to reference the main text because of the idiosyncratic, intuitive and speculative nature of this work. Most of these books referred to will provide bibliographies, so you can pursue your specific areas of interest further.

- A personal *Biography*.

Spellbinding has evolved from an earlier monograph I completed in 2013, called *Just Add Blood*. This shorter descriptive work served to highlight what I believe is a significant focus within the knowledge and use of the runes, or *runelore*; that is, the role of magic and sacrifice.

Symbolically blood is a very powerful vital fluid. In our day and age blood carries a significance that is almost fearful, as we associate it with threatening infectious diseases; yet it can also be life-saving, as with transfusions. Blood is a symbol of power, as indicated in the sacrificial and ritualised acts of many forms of execution. Yet at a deeper spiritual level it is representative of the power of death and transformation, as in the art of alchemy and the blood of the Eucharist. Drawing and using one's own blood is not only a powerful, but also a magical act, and should be approached – and used – with caution; as well as the support of a ritual, ceremony and community, within a spiritual context.

The evolution of my study of runelore since *Just Add Blood* has been sporadic, but intense. I have since left medical practice to focus entirely on my psychospiritual interests, which are associated with or stem from *Just Add Blood* and other works. Leaving medicine was a move that writing this earlier work had a lot to do with, as that exit now feels like an act of initiation. There has been much toil in this period; it has been hard, slow, and not without difficulty. At times, apart from utilising the Futhorc within my ongoing spiritual, therapy and healing work, it has seemed too difficult to pursue in any kind of coherent and meaningful way.

Just Add Blood seemed to have said all that I may be able to contribute to the field. However, the call to do more was and is incessant, and I have felt to respond. *Spellbinding* includes *Just Add Blood* with revision and extension, such that it is unnecessary to read the earlier work prior to engage with *Spellbinding*. This is because I now consider *Just Add Blood* to be an incomplete work and maybe released prematurely, to now be superseded by and included within *Spellbinding*. However, *Just Add Blood* does represent my thinking and relative maturity on the subject at the time, at many levels. Leaving the enmeshment of the medical establishment; able to pursue my ideas unrestricted; and to give my intuition a wider brief, have resulted in a more complete view of the whole field of runelore and magic. It has also allowed me to speculate more broadly and deeply.

It seems relatively obvious to me that runes emerge from deep in pre-history, within whatever priestly caste defined the time, as a tool of communication with the gods or – in modern terminology – the transpersonal or archetypal forces that shape, define and govern our existence. It is no surprise, therefore, that as language and writing emerged for more routine, mundane, and profane means of communication, that runes took a more occult and separate pathway into an esoteric system of communication. They have maintained this position, even if somewhat underground, and it is a source of profound interest to me that they have re-emerged in an age that is decidedly godless.

This means of spiritual communication required and requires various modes, such as appropriate time, location, ritual, and varying degrees of altered states of consciousness. To the informed and observant, the relationship to shamanic tradition is relatively obvious. However, such an orientation usually and necessarily demands a level of sacrifice. In the context here, *Just Add Blood* indicated that the sacrifice was – and is – fundamentally that: The use of the practitioner's own blood from a sacrificial wound embedded into the personally carved, engraved or otherwise shaped runes, within the selected commonly wooden or stone staves that portrayed them. Whilst many might consider such a sacrifice a metaphor and symbolic, there is a level where – like that which occurs in an altered state of consciousness – it is unutterably real.

Having undertaken this rite, *Spellbinding* now offers the next stage in the process.

Introducing the Futhorc

In modern times runes are usually considered within the realms of magic and divination, as well as being a script of sorts. The word rune itself can mean a *secret*, *mystery*, or even a *whisper*. There are differing levels of reality condensed here: Spelling as writing, and *spells* as magic; secrets as things hidden or *occult*, and mystery as things unknown yet also *unknowable*. These different levels pervade our reality, although in modern times there is a tendency to collapse the unknown and unknowable into the known; to reduce the symbolic to the literal, and the magical to the scientific.

My belief is that one significant aspect of the modern attraction to runes is the reconnection with and restoration of this greater mysterious and spiritual reality within a historical tradition and its culture from which we, in modernity, have become largely disconnected. In effect, the runes can exert a *charm*, or magical power. The gods and ancestors are still talking; maybe now we are listening better. Indeed, it could be argued that this reality itself is making itself known through means such as the runes, providing a direct access for us to the gods or spiritual reality in a living manner, and not through the often redundant or closed channels of established religion. It may be that we lose our traditional background and ancestral heritage at our peril, and that one function of runelore is to reverse this process and restore a more holistic and harmonious modern reinstatement. Essentially, I see runelore as a tradition that is integral to human consciousness and its evolution.

In psychospiritual terminology, the Soul is primarily asking for her voice to be heard, and secondly for a reunited path back to the divine. In less mystical or alchemical terms, this is establishing a creative relationship with the greater reality that pervades, permeates, and is inclusive of our mundane existence. This relationship has a language that is necessarily symbolic and imaginative, and not only do the runes fulfil this criterion, it may be that the greater reality itself is using them as a means for getting back in contact with its lost children.

The actual source of the runes is undetermined, although they are ultimately and primarily associated with the Germanic races, which includes modern England, Germany, Holland, Scandinavia and East Germany (formerly the Goths). Whilst the latter is now historical, my personal and intuitive impression is that the Gothic contribution to the runic corpus has not been fully considered. There are other connections, such as the Etruscan (Northern Italian), noted by many as potential source material. It should not be forgotten that the Celts, who preceded the Anglo-Saxons and Romans in Britain, were originally Germanic. I suspect an uninterrupted continuum between the Celts and the Anglo-Saxons, with some intervening Roman infusion, rather than the historical discontinuity that is often implied.

As we gaze back through the British Iron Age that began ~700 BCE (Before the Common Era), considered Celtic and ending with the coming of the Romans in 43 CE, to the Bronze Age beginning ~2,000 BCE and the Neolithic beyond that, there are other considerations to hold in mind. The earliest runes are located in the first centuries of the common era, but what preceded them? What were the influences of other peoples, Celtic and beyond? It is my contention that, as we move backward in time, we approach a more shamanic worldview in which runelore is embedded and emerges from. Although intriguing to me, this area remains speculative. It also has to take into account *Ogham*, the so-called tree alphabet associated with the Celts.

In looking at the known runes, Greek influences may flow through the Gothic channels. The Latin influence appears relatively obvious with some runes, but does not extend to the whole corpus, which probably predates Latin itself. As stated, Etruscan as source material is a currently favoured academic option and is well supported with evidence, including the similarity between some runes and Roman letters. However, the reverse position – that runes may be source material in their own right – is not as generally considered, nor is a parallel development. I wonder whether the prevailing view is a convenient one, in light of the vaster and more nebulous scope of pre-history I have just outlined.

Part of the confusion surrounds the fact that we are so accustomed to the modern alphabet, we do not fully appreciate that there are scripts where the supposed alphabetic letters also have an inherent alternative esoteric meaning. So, when the runic script is explored from a solely literal perspective, it will necessarily be incomplete to our understanding; a kind of proto-script. The Etruscan, Roman, and Greek scripts do not readily have letters with an associated word or symbolic meaning. For example, the Elder Futhark rune ᚠ is the letter *f* and has the name **Fehu**, which means cattle, value, or fee; but the Roman equivalent does not have a similar extension of meanings. So, whilst some Roman letters may have been imported into the runic script, the actual meanings would have been either indigenous to the Germanic peoples, or gained from elsewhere. Maybe a lot of this confusion awaits further evidence and finds, because from a scholarly perspective the available field seems to have been well-tilled to date and any gaps infused with idiosyncratic theories.

There is considerable debate about the time of origin of the runes. The two first centuries of the common era are supported by archaeological evidence and considered the recognised historical minimum. Although, because of the nature of some materials used (wood etc., which would be either naturally or sacrificially destroyed) for which there is no record, an earlier time is widely speculated, even to several hundred years before the common era. Older epigraphic evidence starts to merge with other forms of pictographic expression, as we move backwards in time beyond the common era. So, the reverse view – that the runes emerged from a proto-language and symbolic system that parallels human evolution – is, to my mind, the most likely scenario and would represent a rich source of inquiry. Speech, hand, and eye are maybe more unified and integrated than we routinely consider.

I favour this view when a Celtic–Anglo-Saxon continuum is considered. As already mentioned, the Celts had a script of sorts, known as *Ogham*. Irrespective of the conflicted theories of the origins and usage of Ogham, I see it as a regional and parallel development to the Futhorc that, as we shall see, infuses and informs Ogham with its development in Britain. I also believe that Ogham is a means of communication that may be both literal and symbolic, used in staves or hand signs, and to be shaped by an essentially shamanic culture for ritual, magical, and healing purposes. It would also have been contemporaneous with the early development of the Futhark in Germania. After all, in the modern era, we do have different languages, even dialects, so why cannot the Futhorc and Ogham be similarly considered?

We now move from speculative pre-history into the historical period of the common era. In the period of the early centuries of the common era, the view generally held is that there existed what is now called the Elder Futhark, consisting of 24 runes, which is the basis of study for all practical purposes; it is this that most commentators refer to. The term Futhark is derived from the first six runes (*th* represents one rune, **Thurisaz**), a feature common to all rune systems. The Elder Futhark first definitively appears in the second century CE and was used across the Germanic nations until late in the millennium, when the Roman alphabet gradually superseded it as a script.

This Elder Futhark was present in England after some of the Germanic races (the Angles, Saxons, and Jutes – hereafter referred to collectively as the Anglo-Saxons) migrated to or invaded the south and east of England after the Roman departure early in the 5th century of the CE; although contact, particularly in the north of England, Scotland and Ireland with Scandinavia, would have long been in existence and also less under Roman influence. Based on sea-faring and pre-historical, these contacts have not been adequately considered, in my view. With the Viking expansion of the 9th century, the occupation of much of England in the North and East of England (Northumbria and East Anglia) was under their direct control (the so-called *Danelaw*), leaving only Wessex and parts of Mercia in England as distinctly Anglo-Saxon, or early English.

During this period, the runes underwent some phonetic modification and a progressive extension, with the 4th or *a* rune becoming an *o*, and a (hard) *c* used instead of the *k* of the 6th rune, such that this runic system became referred to as the Anglo-Saxon or Old English *Futhorc*. Note the spelling change of *Futhark* to *Futhorc* as a consequence of this, sometimes via a transitional *Futhork*, which is still occasionally used. As well as other modifications to rune shapes, names, and sounds, there were some additional runes added in England, such that the Futhorc numbers anywhere between the original 24 and 33, or 34 runes. The extension is commonly to 28 or 29 (as in the Old English rune poem), with the last four added later and, interestingly, being peculiar to Northumbria.

What I find interesting about this extension is that it starts to go beyond what is the necessary number required for a language system; ours is now set at 26 in Modern English, for example. This sets the Futhorc apart, in my thinking, particularly as there is also some tentative and obscure further extension occurring in the medieval period proper; that is, after 1066. It is my contention that these developments encompass a mystical trend – symbolic and initiatory – as marked by alchemy and, later in the medieval period, the Grail legends. To these themes, we will return.

In Scandinavia, the Elder Futhark underwent a radical revision and reduction during the Viking era (800 – 1100 CE approx.) from 24 to 16 runes, and subsequently became referred to as the *Younger Futhark*. The reasons for this are unclear, but may mark a possible division between magico-mystical purposes and the usage of runes as a simple script, as well as an attempt to re-establish a more traditional religious autonomy in the face of advancing Christianity.

The Roman script progressively predominated during this entire period (400-1100 CE approx.), generally contemporaneous with the Christianisation of Northern Europe. The runes then relatively disappear from public view after the Norman invasion of England in 1066 and the close of the Viking era around 1100, with sporadic appearances over the second millennium – mainly in folklore and magical channels – culminating in the modern resurgence of interest. It should not be forgotten that the Normans, although from France, were originally Norsemen from Scandinavia.

Common materials for carving runes include wood (there are many and frequent references to trees in all of the Futharks), bone (possibly ritualistic), coins (generally from the middle of the first millennium), epigraphic (on stones), and also in manuscripts (usually Christian). (Please note: *Futharks* is a collective term referring to all three rune-rows – the Elder Futhark, Younger

Futhark and the Futhorc.) Whilst stone runes occur predominantly in Scandinavia, interestingly there is a cluster in northern rather than southern England, often in religious settings and possibly reflecting the ongoing Norse and Viking influences.

Other sources of information include the rune poems. The Old English rune poem dates from the 8th to the 9th century, written by Christian scribes from earlier sources. The original poem was destroyed by a fire in the 18th century, but an earlier accurately acknowledged copy exists. This poem describes 29 runes. The Scandinavian Younger Futhark is referred to in two poems recorded in the 13th (Norway) and 15th centuries (Iceland), also from Christian sources. There is, unfortunately and interestingly, no equivalent poem for the Elder Futhark. The English rune poem is often referred to for understanding the Elder Futhark, although modified by the Younger Futhark rune poems (obviously, this is only possible for 16 of the 24 runes). This may represent an attempt, by some commentators, to gain a clearer or more original and authentic meaning from the Germanic perspective, as there are several significant differences in the poems.

These are the basic facts, but what are the varied reasons that stand behind them? Here we meet a mixture of knowledge, opinion and speculation over a very wide spectrum.

The more academic and scholarly position (as with RI Page, particularly with regard to the English Futhorc) is generally literal and mundane and posits that runes represent a script for various purposes, such as communication, legal documents, possession of property, and epigraphs. This position eschews a primarily religious or magical dimension, and indeed the evidence as such does not overtly and directly support one; although it is problematic to consider how it could.

Yet the circumstantial evidence seems overwhelming, plus the fact that the modern alphabet and runic scripts appear side by side in many finds, indicating that the latter were used for a fundamentally different purpose. However, as with other disciplines – modern western medicine, for example in my experience – a strict scientific and evidence-based methodology does not include more speculative and intuitive approaches, and would also tend to deny the existence of a magico-religious influence by exclusion, repression, and literalisation.

Here is where I part company with the strict scholarly approach. I am not alone in this: RWV Elliott retains a sound scholarly background in the Futhorc, yet does cross the divide into the magico-religious. Nigel Pennick adds considerable insight and depth to the Futhorc and explores the extensions beyond the 29 of the rune poem. Edred Thorsson has a PhD in this academic domain and champions a modern Germanic magico-religious view around runelore and the Futhark. Others, such as Kveldulf Gundarsson, have followed Thorsson in the Germanic domain (both are from a North American background), as well as Freya Aswynn and Jan Fries in Europe. The varied input of JRR Tolkien has, in my opinion, yet to be thoroughly assessed in this context.

Interestingly, the Anglo-Saxon Futhorc gets a more psycho-social orientation (for example, by Alaric Albertsson, also a North American), in line with the apparent trend in the Futhorc away from the more magico-religious view present in the Elder Futhark. Indeed, and as I have already indicated, it could be argued (and is by the likes of Thorsson) that the development of the Younger Futhark in the Viking era was to maintain or even re-establish these magico-religious dimensions in the advance of the more literal Roman script and alphabet, as well as dealing with any Christian repression. However, and as will be discussed, whilst this psycho-social orientation in the Futhorc obviously exists, it does not exclude the magico-religious one that I believe occurs at least within the so-called rune extension.

Of interest is that in England there was the continued use of epigraphic stone runes in the North during the latter part of the first millennium of the CE. It is possible that the Christian Church in the North had a different view of runes and, being more distant from the Roman Church's influence, tended to be more holistic and integrative of other views and beliefs. The Church in the north was also somewhat idiosyncratic, as with the views of the Celtic Christian Pelagius in the 5th century, as well as issues around tonsures and the dating of Easter that were raised at the Synod of Whitby in the 7th century, where the Roman Church finally gained the upper hand over the Celtic Church.

Northern England, Scotland and Ireland were also the sites of Viking contact from the early 9th century, so their influence of the development of the Younger Futhark may also have been significant from at least that time, and probably before. Trade in the North between England and Scandinavia existed well before this time, which is hardly surprising for a seafaring power able to reach Iceland, Greenland and North America many centuries before Columbus in the 15th century.

However, and in general, there was an increasing use of the Roman script within these societies during this period, such that the Old English language becomes and is now referred to entirely in Roman script. There were a couple of included anomalies, as with the retention of the runes **Thorn** – ᚦ – for **th** and **Wyn** – ᚹ – for **w**, with occasional others where there is some degree of overlap between the two systems. This would obviously have been a progressive, regional, and varied development. Although these runic inclusions have now been excluded from our modern language, they are frequently retained in Old English studies. It is of interest to me that whilst the Roman script was retained, Latin as a tongue was not: Old English has become the source of the language that dominates the globe, with its source in Indo-

European via the Germanic languages, specifically the Anglo-Saxon tongue.

A little tangentially, it may be of value to sketch out a very rough and somewhat speculative timeline of the development of the runes. To do this in any further depth and increased comprehension demands evidence from other fields (historical, archaeological, mythological etc.), as well as an understanding of the influence of religion and politics over the same period.

What I propose here is that the runes had, what could be called, a proto-runic history that extends back in time, possibly at least until the end of the last Ice Age, about 10,000 BCE. Various markings in places like caves have distinctly runic elements, although the majority are either only vaguely similar, or quite dissimilar. It is not difficult to postulate these markings and their development as expressions of a humanity making sense of itself and the world, as well as trying to communicate this in various ways. The imaginative, creative, shamanic and magical influences of this would have been strong.

This may explain the apparent Gothic and Etruscan influences, as well as their relationship to other similar systems (such as the Roman script), as the Elder Futhark emerged as a kind of common system, or written language of sorts. We are now in the early part of the Common Era. This seems to be what emerged in Britain during this period from the Germanic world, interestingly at around the same time that Christianity's influence was arriving and overlapping it via the Roman Empire. Added to this is meeting the indigenous Celtic system of Ogham, purportedly that of the priestly class, or Druids, marking the beginnings of the Futhorc and the subsequent inclusion of several runes – 25 to 27 – with the seeming distinct influence of Ogham, as well as with some emergence into a common system.

Speculatively, **Ior**, rune 28, could have a similar function to the final rune, **Gar**, as some sort of overall map of the Futhorc, including its primal association with the serpent, worm, or ouroboros. And, although **Ear**, rune 29, is included in the Old English rune poem, it appears to me to be more in keeping with the four latter runes, 30 to 33, called Northumbrian by virtue of origin. These runes were added later in the first millennium when the Christian influence was increasing and Northumbria was a bastion of Celtic influences in the religious mix. As we will come to, these runes have a more esoterically Christian flavour to them.

However, the runes, after an apparent period of co-existence with the Roman script of Latin, were subsequently overshadowed by it. From this point, their prominence and influence appear to diminish and sink into the undercurrents of history, with occasional resurfacing and even some addition to the rune sequence that we will return to.

The Roman influence seems to have won the day and this was reinforced by the events of 1066 and with what followed. Britain generally, and England specifically, was now on a different course. Roman influence may have failed militarily, but its religion eventually seized the day. This is reflected politically, where the separation between Church and State is not how we would have it today. It is also present in other fields; for example, where Mediterranean medicine won out against the indigenous Heathen variety, in spite of its later Christianisation. However, I am careful about extending too far with military terminology, as all these processes are far more fluid and cohesive than maybe we have given credit for.

As a brief aside: I adopt the word *heathen*, rather than *pagan*, throughout; in brief, because the former is a Germanic word and the latter Roman. In this way, the rather derogatory and pejorative way the word *pagan* is commonly used is given a bit of psychic distance. Derived from the word for uncultivated open land, or *heath*, I find Heathen a little more poetic and descriptive.

I have also chosen to capitalise it, so that the word Heathen is on a par with Christian.

I contend that the more esoteric view of runes is ultimately shamanic; this position being exemplified by Woden in a symbolic manner (see later text). This is in spite of the modern revival of Druidry – a somewhat aristocratic class of Celtic priesthood – that is probably over-emphasised because of ongoing and political awkwardness about any Germanic spiritual revivalism. There is a tendency toward a sanitised view of Old English spirituality as being predominantly Celtic. I consider this inaccurate and creating an unnecessary distortion. Moreover, other commentators have tried to reinstate Germanic shamanism as a fundamental tradition in England. Brian Bates (a university academic with a PhD) has done this in *The Way of Wyrd* and, even though the work itself is fictional, it is based on scholarly evidence derived from the *Lacnunga*, a miscellaneous text of remedies, prayers and charms written in the late tenth century from prior oral tradition.

As a further aside, Druidry is commonly associated with the Celts in Britain, although the Celtic migrations, also from the Germanic regions, occurred quite late (around 700-500 BCE). Druids are thus of the emerging Iron Age and have nothing directly to do with the Stone Age culture that produced monuments like Stonehenge, at least two thousand years earlier. Druidry may have continuity with older priestly classes that existed prior to the Celtic migrations, but ultimately its structure and power were decimated by the Roman invasion of North-western Europe. Any survival may have been assimilated within the Anglo-Saxon culture and also become progressively Christianised.

That this shamanic influence is less obvious in England than elsewhere in Northern Europe is probably partly due to the initial

Roman influence, as England was the only country in our exploration that was colonised in this period. There was also the influence of Christianity early in the Anglo-Saxon period of occupation, formally at the turn of the 7th century, though existent well prior within the Roman occupation, following their own conversion in the 4th century.

Christianity did not reach the northern lands until much later in the millennium. This was a progressive movement, with Iceland converting democratically in 1000 CE. However, Scandinavia was a more mixed affair with conversion in some regions being even later than Iceland, around the 12th century. Even with this conversion, which was often for political reasons on behalf of the indigenous authorities and hence more token, the religious undercurrent in Germanic cultures remained strongly Heathen. It doesn't take much imagination to see the trends here with this explanation, nor that the Viking influence – including their spirituality – was more significant than has been previously recognised, particularly in the North and East of England.

This is not to minimise the significant and dominant influence of the Christian Church from at least a political and social perspective. Christianity has ended up the victor in this domain, although the current runic revival indicates some sort of psychological redress. It is well known that the Church had a repressive position toward religions and spiritual positions that were not in conformity with it, such that in our current predominantly Christian society this perspective, and its inherent distortions, still holds sway. That there is a divide between the academic and esoteric positions has not been further helped by the sometimes extreme and highly speculative positions held by many of the latter in the public domain, particularly those of so-called New Age persuasion.

From a more spiritual perspective, all languages are ultimately seen to be associated with the *word* of the gods or God. Woden (Odin in Scandinavia, Wodan or Wotan in Germany) is often seen as the most significant god in the northern pantheon, although historically this has not always been so, as both Tyr and Thor had considerable and sometimes prior and later influence, respectively. Woden is also the god of ecstasy (a shamanic feature) and poetry (the word). His self-sacrifice and discovery of the runes, as described in the *Havamal* (sourced in the Poetic Edda of the Viking era: See appendix) is distinctly shamanic, as well as having clear symbolic overtones to the crucifixion and resurrection, which I am sure attracted the repressive tendencies of the Church. One consequence of his ordeal was the expression of eighteen charms or spells that have mythological and runic significance.

Personally, I wonder whether it is correct to view Woden as a god, he appears more as a shaman or magician here – with similarities to the Celtic Merlin – and with Christ-like features that may pose a greater threat than simply and conveniently viewing him as a primitive Heathen god. He also seems to have emerged and consolidated his spiritual position as the era progressed, with a significant Viking boost to his status. This very condensed picture of Woden can be seen to have all sorts of ramifications regarding northern spirituality generally, including shamanism, and the runes in particular.

This can be further exemplified in discussing some of the idiosyncrasies in the various rune rows. In the Elder Futhark, the 4th rune is called **Ansuz** and is considered as a god (commonly Odin or Wodan) on interpretation. By the time we get to the English Futhorc, the rune has become **Os** and, whilst sometimes referring generically to a god (specifically Woden), it is commonly interpreted as a mouth, although – maybe somewhat ironically – this could be seen as Woden's poetic side. Similarly, the 3rd rune

Thurisaz can be the god *Thor* or a giant in the Futhark, whilst in the Futhorc it becomes **Thorn** – a *thorn*. The additional runes in the Futhorc also have names that are associated with trees (oak, ash), beyond those (birch, yew) common to the other two Futharks, as well as materials and elements (stone, fire, earth) and products (spear, bow) that are more practical and maybe not only just for mundane usage and communication. These trends I consider both interesting and important.

The 6th rune in the Elder Futhark is **Kenaz**, which can relate to an ulcer or a sore. There are further shamanic associations here – as well as some sexual ones – with wounding, sacrifice and healing. In the Futhorc, this rune becomes **Cen** and the meaning, a *torch*. The 22nd rune **Ing** changes meaning from the northern god Ing to simply the sound *ng* in the Futhorc. Once again, there is a demythologisation process apparent, but a further irony could be that this last rune – **Ing** – could be one source of the country named England; intriguing to consider the country may be named after a Heathen god!

Of course, that many runes refer to details such as the day, year, and sun, is no great surprise with the agricultural lifestyle and climatic conditions of the north. The seasons and their magical mastery, and possibly the significance of ritual and ceremonies contained in all the Futharks, point to a magical and spiritual relationship to and with the land. Also, the references to animals are clear, even including the now-extinct aurochs (a large and wild breed of ox or bison). Although it is interesting that, beyond the serpent in the expanded Futhorc, there is no reference to birds or water species of animal; even the serpent could relate to the mythic worm, or a dragon. There is also no reference to mythic animals or beings, nor is there any reference to supernatural beings or forces beyond the individual gods themselves.

I also find the absence of direct reference to metals interesting in an era that follows the bronze and iron ages; is this because the runes are even more ancient than we have assumed to date? There is a reference to a spear, but not a sword. Does this reinforce the rhetorical nature of the above question, or might the last Futhorc runes of *chalice*, *stone*, and *spear* refer to other functions? The spear is present in both the crucifixion (sometimes) and Odin's self-sacrifice. The stone is both an alchemical concept and associated with King-making. The chalice, seemingly connected to Christianity and maybe a borrowed term from Celtic folklore, may also hark back to the use of the drinking horn. There are echoes here of the Arthurian corpus and the spiritual significance of the Holy Grail, which is also an alchemical motif. There are no rune poems to clarify these issues, yet they remain tantalising.

Other meanings are generally mundane and practical, at one level, though they can have a deeper more metaphoric meaning if a more esoteric perspective is taken; which is how the rune poems should be approached, in my opinion. From the mundane and physical levels, runic meanings can extend to the sexual, cultural, social, psychological, mythic, and spiritual domains. The possibilities seem endless, but isn't this a fundamental quality of symbolism?

Runes are presented as a pictograph, an associated letter (of the Roman alphabet, when considered literally), a name, sound, and a meaning. There may be several of these meanings within each rune, possibly due to levels of kenning in the rune-master and the context in which the runes are used. In general, I will not be taking a literal approach to the runes, as the alphabet associations – although academically and otherwise interesting – do not directly further the more symbolic and magical perspectives, so these will be used only as necessary.

Consideration should not be lost on the pictographic aspect

itself; the runes should be seen primarily as symbols in their own right, an expression of evolving consciousness perhaps? The aurochs is a wild and powerful beast: Is the shape of the **Ur** rune in the Futharks – an inverted **U** or ᚢ – that of the beast with the head down and horns protruding? For those of a more Freudian persuasion, the sexual aspects may stick out (pun intended). In fact, many of the runes lend themselves to not only sexual interpretation, but also to hand gestures and bodily positions for either one or two people: A western yoga and Tantra perhaps?

This is the first spectrum that needs to be considered; from literal to metaphoric, and then to the symbolic, incorporating names and meanings. But also, there is another parallel perspective that I will arbitrarily define as psychological, divinatory, and magical. Psychological refers to the meaning that is commonly represented within the rune, and is the basis for the next two perspectives. The divinatory is when the runes are consulted in response to a query or question; that is, when the spiritual is being asked to intercede in mundane reality (this could be loosely equated with praying). The magical approach is when the rune-master (magician or shaman) uses the runes to effect change in reality, through active magical intercession in the spiritual domains.

A divinatory approach involves a reading, or layout of runes, generally in response to a query. A common method is to draw – unseen – from the rune-pouch three runes, in succession. The first representing what underlays the query (*past*), the second where the querent or rune-master presently stands with the query (*present*), and the third what the query is portending (*future*). My preference for other words than past etc. indicates that the time factor here should be considered fluid and relative, and not in the linear and fixed manner we currently perceive it, otherwise we can get tangled up and confused with concepts like fate and free will. It is probable the Germanic peoples also saw time in a similar and more cyclic manner.

In the divinatory method, not only should the runes be read psychologically in an individual sense, but the overall pattern appreciated and interpreted. This orientation is expanded in one magical approach, where a so-called bindrune (usually a combination of two, three or more runes-into-one) is used for the purposes of a charm or spell. In this case, the runemaster may select the runes to be used and commit them to a ritual process to effect change. However, there are many more varied approaches that can – obviously – be used here and would have been relatively secret; which is another reason why the bequeathed runic material does not easily lend itself to a magical interpretation.

To gain a further appreciation of these various areas, the writers referred to in the bibliography should be explored. Other approaches that would be useful include the fields of shamanism and the magical disciplines. I must state here, as an Englishman by birth, that one imbalance I am trying to redress is the preference in magical circles, from just over one hundred years ago, towards symbolic systems (such as the Tarot), languages (such as Hebrew), and magical systems (such as the Kabbalah) that may not resonate with the northern mentality. Nor might any casual indirect reference to Freud (via sexuality); Jung may be a better option, with his symbolic appreciation, mystical outlook, and theory of archetypes that approach *the gods*. Of possible associated interest is that Freud was an Austrian Jew, and Jung a Swiss of Germanic descent.

Taking a psychoanalytic perspective on the concept of repression one step further, and beyond my comments above about the sexual interpretations: What does the modern revival have to tell us?

I suspect the modern revival is just that, a *return of the repressed* in psychoanalytic parlance, which includes sexuality anyway; although a more Jungian perspective would be of more intellectual, expansive, and creative interest. The argument would go like this: We have been psychically separated from these deeper spiritual aspects of ourselves by the repressive and controlling forces within Christianity, as well as by other associated cultures. Whilst this may have suited the political and power ambitions within northern society at the time, it has and does not lead to a longer-term more holistic integration, and thus our present confused position with respect to our indigenous spirituality. Even the events in 20th century Germany should be seen in this light, if properly viewed from a creative, as well as the more commonly perceived destructive and often prejudiced perspective.

Consequently, there is a psychological imperative to get beyond this repression and to reconnect with these deep forces. These could be considered archetypal in Jung's terms, but to consider the Heathen gods as simply archetypes, in some sort of psychological reductionism, would be a grave error: The gods are not simply archetypes. Instead, we should see them as vital forces within and beyond the individual subjective psyche, or soul, that demand a hearing and can demand a reintegration: We ignore them at our peril. If your disposition is fundamentally Germanic, then the runes would be a valid pathway for this exploration and reunification ... they could be *for you.*

The overall understanding of runelore is of gaining a connection, a relationship, to the greater psychic reality in which we are embedded. A fundamental is that this reality is all-powerful, wise, and knowing, as in the Christian sense of God. It is also eternal and infinite, such that the present contains all the spectrum of our past and future. Yet we are an expression of this greater reality in time and space, and in some mysterious way involved in its – our – evolution and consciousness.

The language of this relationship I contend is deeply imaginative and expressed symbolically. Hence the complexity of the runes, comprising levels of image, sound, name and meaning in a multi-faceted manner that can be seen as such a language and transcending less complete systems. This complexity is fundamentally holistic ranging from the known to the mysterious, recognising that human understanding is possible, but limited. Beyond this is a step into gnosis ...

The Anglo-Saxon Mentality

Before we engage the Futhorc directly, I would like to provide a perspective of the Anglo-Saxon mindset; because it differs from our modern one in some significant ways, even though there are considerable areas of overlap. I would also like to identify this mindset with a more immanent sense of the soul than we commonly appreciate in the modern era. Generally, it appears the soul was more immediately apprehended, as compared to the modern notion of it, where it is usually seen in a more distant and transcendent manner.

Modern psychology has adopted the word *Self* as a kind of hub around which the various components of our experience satellite in some sort of individualistic manner. In many ways, I can see the usefulness of this term, but I think that can become confused with the term, *Ego*, as well as being a statement about our modern hyper-individualised mentality. I also believe that *Self* detracts from the connections that the individual has to the more objective or transpersonal psyche and hence to spirit, so is a major reason I favour and champion the term *Soul*. The term *Self* is better reserved for our space and linear time bound-being in the world, and so intimately connected with our cognition, senses, instincts and the body generally.

I see the *Soul* as a more inclusive concept around which to centre our life experience with its intrapsychic experience, emotional fluidity, cyclical nature and connection to the broader psychic reality, including the spiritual. Although I am profoundly influenced by Jungian ideas, I am not using *Self* the way he or other Jungians allude to, but in the more restricted manner described above. Jung would see his term to unify all aspects of the psyche, being collective as well as personal, so reflective of a spirit-soul continuum.

In the modern era, we take a physical and biomechanical orientation, first and foremost. The *Mind* is considered to be some sort of by-product of the physical organ called the brain. The functions of the mind are often seen in a limited cognitive manner and operating in specific ways, such as causally, reductively, and quantitatively. This sort of perspective we often refer to with the Greek *Psyche* that, even though it translates to *Soul*, is a word we tend to use more for this rational mind, around which we position irrational components in a way that we mistakenly assume will one day become identified and understood by neuroscience, as well as behavioural, research, and academic psychology; that is, they will become cognitively understood and hence rational.

We have come to a lot of confusion with a mixture of English, Greek and Latin terms; different schools of Psychology, and even the input of other disciplines such as modern physics. In this earlier Anglo-Saxon era, that confusion was by no means the case: The body and mind were seen as a fundamental although complex unity of a more holistic nature, with the concern being more for the soul and a far emotionally richer concept than our modern worldview of psyche – a term not then known or used, of course.

I generally try to avoid using the word *Psyche* because it is commonly used in a rational, cognitive and modern context as equivalent to *Mind*. In fact, I prefer the noun *Mentality* to *Psyche* for these reasons, within this modern context. If I do use *Psyche*, it is in a more mythic and/or depth psychological (Jungian) manner. My inclination is to use it in two ways: a subjective and personal psyche inclusive of the body, roughly equivalent to the *Soul*; or an objective one, more equivalent to the transpersonal world we recognise as *Spirit*. This concept of psyche is even greater than that of the soul, so making its modern reduction and limitation to the rational mind counter-productive and problematic, to my way of thinking.

When I use the words *psychic* or *psychically* as adjectives or adverbs, they are descriptive and should be seen as equivalent to this broader concept of psyche, that includes our personal or subjective experience, but also approaches the spiritual realms. *Mental* or *mentally* are the equivalents for the rational mind and the thinking process in daily reality, or realm of the *Self* as I define it inclusive of the body. I retain the *psych-* prefix, when appropriate. The astute observer will not be surprised to hear that I find the disciplines of psychology and psychiatry quite problematic from a nominal perspective!

To avoid many of these difficulties, I will refer to the *Soul* directly as I understand it, and as described above. This is more compatible with the Anglo-Saxon Mentality than with modern views, which is a reason to consider that mentality in more detail here. This appreciation of the soul sees it – commonly seen as her – as more of a process than a structure, emotionally-laden, and having a primary creative or imaginal function. The soul extends to other varied facets of the broader psyche, as in *psychoerotic, psychospiritual* or *psychosocial*, which is another reason to retain the *psych-* prefix, though not to reduce these terms to the rational mind exclusively.

Finally, in this aside, I will be briefly mentioning a couple of perspectives that I will be taking a different slant on, or avoiding altogether. Firstly gender, which I will be approaching as psychic principles of masculinity and femininity, common to both men and women. The relationship of these principles to their physical manifestation in the sexes is problematic and I believe we still have a long way to go in picturing this more realistically and creatively, which I do elsewhere in my writings. In this study, I will be referring to masculinity and femininity as principles in a more archetypal context, better described by disciplines such as mythology.

Secondly, I will avoid using the words *conscious* and *consciousness*, particularly when they refer to or imply the opposite of the *unconscious*. If gender is manifestly problematic, I find this the more subtly so. It creates the impression of the unclearly defined term *Self* being the authority in matters psychic and spiritual, and leads to all sorts of distortions. It becomes a dangerous tool in rhetoric, interpersonal relationships and disciplines like psychiatry. *Unconscious* is best avoided; because, if other simpler words and expressions can be used, they circumnavigate the judgmental dangers inherent in its usage; most particular is the tendency in some areas to somehow equate it with God.

In contrast to our modern perspective, largely influenced by Christian theology, the Anglo-Saxon mentality was of a unified complex of various entities that included the body. The body, like the mind and other non-physical features of the individual, is seen as included within this *Soul* or *Body-Soul Complex*. By contrast in the modern era, we tend to see the soul as some sort of separate entity in the body, commonly located in the head, and something like a homunculus. Christianity would potentially find more favour with this latter perspective for various reasons.

A distinguishing feature of the modern Christian view is that the soul is primarily a spiritual component of the Godhead, consequently separate from the physical body, and also the individual self. There are, obviously, all sorts of consequences to this view that essentially render the soul distant from the physically experiencing self, and only contactable through the Church and its teachings. This was to become an emergent position, not nearly as evident in the first millennium of the CE, and has much to do with politics and social control, as we are increasingly coming to realise.

But for the Heathen there was – is – no such separation. The soul, with all its facets, is seen to connect with and include the body, at one end of a spectrum or simply as an entity amongst others. At the other end of this spectrum, its increasingly ephemeral and less personal facets merge into the world of spirit. This world houses the gods and goddesses, the elves and dwarves, the spirit of plant and animal, ghosts and spectres, and is expressed in a rich mythology and cosmology. Because of the much earlier influence of Christianity in Britain, this richness in it is not as evident, which is one reason we need to draw on other related systems of belief in the broader Germanic world.

It would also be wrong to see the coming together of the indigenous Heathen worldview with that of Christianity as some sort of competition and psychological warfare; a view unfortunately held by many of modern pagan communities. As we will come to, even the later runes of the Futhorc indicate a dialectic and creative fusion at the mystical levels of alchemy, as well as maybe being a precursor to the later Grail legends. The Celtic Church preceded the more formal Roman version for some centuries up to and maybe until the Synod of Whitby in 664 CE. Interestingly, Whitby is in the English North, in Northumbria, whose influence on the Futhorc was quite marked, particularly in the runes of mystical interest.

Embedded in the symbolism of the Germanic peoples are some surprisingly modern concepts. The image of Woden, the shamanic god of the Anglo-Saxon, who is minus an eye that he sacrificed in the attainment of the runes and wisdom, reminds us of the equivalent opening of inner wisdom or the so-called *third eye*. This image, or similar, is present in many cultural myths. But, pertinent here, is that two ravens sat – or sit – on Woden's shoulders, one representing thought, the other memory. This knowledge they would find in their world travels and whisper in Woden's ear; whisper, it will be recalled, is also a reference to the word *rune*.

Thought (in Old English – OE – *hyge*) is information gathering (via the raven) and reasoning, retrieved from memory. It is associated with perception, cognition and the will, or intention. In general, it is the processing of unrefined information. In Old English *hyge* is a masculine noun. In modern neurophysiology, these are the functions that we associate with the left cerebral hemisphere, or the so-called colloquial *masculine brain*. It approximates considerably to the concept of the mind in modernity.

By contrast mind (OE *mynd* or *gemynd*) is memory of learned knowledge and wisdom, the personal memories accumulated in the individual's lifetime. Yet there is also a deeper level of memory that is instinctual or inborn, approaching ancestral memory. *Mynd* is a feminine noun and here associated with the right cerebral hemisphere, or the so-called colloquial *feminine brain*. The associations and symbolism embedded here, even down to some of the Old English words, are appreciable.

Emotion (OE *mod*) is given a more unifying quality and one that elevates its importance and significance than we now more commonly appreciate, although some significant commentators – myself included – have sought to redress this imbalance. The very name *mod* suggests mood. Its usage here is more than mere emotion, in the physiological sense; it refers to related qualities and values, such as honour and integrity, and can be seen more as the heart in a metaphoric sense. I believe the role of emotion and mood in memory is presently understated and not well understood, mainly because of the cognitive perspective of the mind we now undertake. Neurophysiologically, *mod* represents the limbic system or, somewhat appropriately, the mid-brain. It also connects functionally more with the right cerebral hemisphere than the left. Paradoxically, this better approximates the soul as I see it, particularly when its connections to emotion are considered.

Combined with the intellect, *mod* moves beyond the dualism of subjectivity and objectivity into a psychic reality, which modern neurophysiological research into shamanism is also beginning to recognise. Feasibly these states bring us to ecstasy, divine madness and inspiration, all features of the shaman, magician and Woden. What to call this in Modern English may be problematical, but not so to the Anglo-Saxon, who recognised it as *wod* and hence Woden. The root *od* in Germanic culture generally refers to ecstasy, or a high state of enthusiasm, as well as being defining of the Woden-related Germanic god, the Norse *Odin*.

The related word *ond* in Germanic culture refers to the life-breath, which gives life to the body-soul complex that has matured through gestation, and is considered to occur several days after birth. It is also a gift of Odin (Woden) and, intuitively, nestled in these concepts is the so-called *divine spark* that connects the body-soul to the spiritual world. The breaking of this bond, if temporary, may reflect the magician-shaman's flight into the world of spirit and, if permanent, death ensues; the soul departs and the body degenerates.

In some senses, the above can be considered more personal and physical. I believe that this psychic reorientation is sufficient to provide a view of the Anglo-Saxon mindset that is not that unfamiliar to the modern one, if a little creative latitude is allowed. I also think that adopting this revised mindset will put you, the reader, in a better position to understand the runes and hence how to use them.

Beyond these features of the personal soul are the more spiritual ones that connect with or reside in the body-soul complex, but that extend to the more transpersonal world of spirit. Following the section on the individual runes, we will have cause to reconnect to the soul as it ventures into the realms of spirit. This exploration will be better understood and appreciated by first looking at the Futhorc runes through the eyes of the Anglo-Saxon soul.

How to Use the Runes

Firstly, a personal note: There are several reasons for my choice of the Futhorc. The first is my English background, reinforced by the fact that for most of us Modern English is our language of choice, which connects directly with the Old English language that supervened the runes, using Latin script. The rune poems begin chronologically with the Old English rune poem, if the written medium is considered. This is source material for the Futhorc and is inclusive of the Elder Futhark, because the latter has no corresponding poem, which I find an interesting fact.

I have found that magical exploration of the later Younger Futhark to be of value. I have opted in the past to use the Elder Futhark for divinatory purposes in my work with other people, as most commentators seem to have done, and still do. I then gravitated to the Futhorc, which has more psycho-social significance for me and is also expressive of my personal heritage. I am currently exploring the relevance of the whole Futhark runic system from the perspective of living in Australia.

As an Englishman, now permanently resident in Australia, I see that this exploration can serve other functions. Europeans still have an uneasy relationship with the Australasian continent and particularly its spirituality. Aboriginal culture may be of value, but is probably not the only avenue for ex-patriot Europeans to examine in making Australia their spiritual home. Instead, I believe we need to explore our own indigenous spirituality and bring this to bear on living in Australia. In one sense, this present exploration of runelore could be seen as a beginning that could extend to deeper psychological, mythological, and cosmological perspectives, as yet unknown.

Introduction

I find *How To...* books a bit of an anomaly. I always wonder how far instruction can be provided in book form, when beyond a certain point education demands more verbal, ritual and initiatory perspectives. In this respect, I am under no illusion, so I generally buy books for their intellectual and informative value, then adapt these to my own personal development and evolutionary process. In general, I find *how to* books to be simplistic, and sometimes both inflated and arrogant; beyond a certain point I ask myself, how the author can possibly claim such authority?

Yet we are an evolving species, information exchange is both rapid and extensive. As I sit here writing I can draw upon a dictionary, as well as spellcheck, go online to confirm facts, and surf to follow associations and other lines of thinking that arise as I write. I can draw on a font for the runes, and can reach out and refer to books from my collection that I may have sourced and received from overseas in a matter of days. I can phone, text, email, or engage colleagues online in a variety of formats for discussion and information. We literally live in a *New Age*, so I ask myself what a genuine *how to* book may look like in this context and time?

Certainly, in my own background I have a significant educational, training and initiatory development in the intellectual, professional and spiritual fields. This comprises written education, but also lectures, seminars, workshops, personal therapy, spiritual instruction, rites of passage, life experience and more ... it is in this context that I see the runes. I most certainly do not see them in the way many would use the horoscope in the paper, as just some sort of simplistic guide for the day.

But firstly, why the runes? My belief is that any magical system must draw the individual to and into it. There are a range of such systems available, probably the most common and familiar being the Tarot and the I Ching. All are derived from Tradition (I am using the capital here pointedly) and hence have the capacity to resonate within the individual at levels beyond their personal narrative, particularly if a more racial and collective viewpoint of inheritance is taken. During the course of my personal development, I have researched and practised with all these tools, but it was the runes that drew me in.

But what does it mean to be *drawn in*? My initial experience was that runes seemed to respond more than other methods to my divinatory questions; it was as if a dialogue with an unknown person or reality was occurring. And the more I communicated, the deeper the dialogue became. This continued for quite a period, although I was very reluctant to use the runes – or anything for that matter – for actual operative magic. I surmised that the runes were a part of my heritage, and this has proven to be the case. I also started to *see* things in a runic way in everyday life, and individual runes started to appear in my dreams.

I would imagine that most of you reading this are in a similar position, although of varying levels of exposure and personal development. Beyond using the runes for personal amusement (when they may not communicate to you in a meaningful manner anyway), I believe their exploration should be in the context of a broad personal developmental approach to life, in whatever form that takes. Mine has been most varied, eclectic, and somewhat erratic at times … but that also suits my disposition.

Yet it is inevitable that this approach would translate into my orientation as to *how to* … The governing disciplines in this, for me, are depth psychology, alchemy, shamanism and magic (in no particular order). As a former holistic medical practitioner with a predominantly mental health psychotherapeutic practice, this orientation suited both my personal and professional lives. From a Jungian background, I see myself as a post-Jungian exploring the analytic and depth psychologies in an eclectic manner. Alchemy is a discipline I believe has a wide and as yet unexplored application to mental and physical health. Shamanism, in the modern context of a more *freestyle* shamanism, is drawing upon whatever disciplines and approaches suit my disposition. Similarly with magic, where a freestyle approach may be the modern term that best applies, and for which the runes are my primary tool in the operative sense.

Yes, I have stepped into and practice operative magic, and this *how to…* will guide you to this position. However, beyond a certain point you are on your own, hence some of my earlier comments about personal experience and development. In this respect, I can only provide an educative background and guidance to this point for each reader individually, which will be governed by your personal development and maturity. Beyond that you are on your own, although maybe with the help and guidance of a mentor.

And this is how I have tried to write this particular book of runelore, to date. I have left a lot out, partly because there is much missing that may never be retrieved, also partly because some of the dots I have joined up are instruction, leaving gaps for you to join others to suit your own disposition. But mainly because that is the nature of the beast; it is a vast jigsaw with some constellations, a lot of gaps, as well as having a border that has not yet and may never be been defined.

I will try and be progressive from the educative position I have outlined to date. Initially my approach will be instructive and relatively simple, but as we progress the process will overtake any structure and become more fluid. At some point, and progressively thereafter, your own experience will come increasingly to the fore. Any ideas and intuitions you may have are totally valid, as working with a system that is greater than your own will guide you increasingly, in the spiritual sense.

You may get to a point in this *how to…* section where you need my, or any other guidance, no longer; and that is totally valid. So, let's step into this vast sea …

Getting to know the Runes

Have you got a rune set? If you have, it is most likely to be one of the Elder Futhark; check by counting the numbers and comparing the images. One guide is the 6th rune of **Cen/Kenaz/Kaun**, which is different in each of three rune rows of the Futharks. Because I am working with the extended 33 rune Futhorc, then try to obtain a longer rune version (28, 29 or 33); however, working with the Elder Futhark will suffice for the time being.

It may be a little early to make your own, but if not here, ultimately it is the thing to do; particularly if you find the runes talk to you, and certainly if you are going to use them for operative magic. You may end up with more than one set and possibly use them for different purposes. But in the meantime, there is the creative possibility of drawing and sketching them, and so familiarising yourself in this manner. One immediate creative possibility is to obtain or make some oblong or circular blank cards (like playing cards) or small stones, and sketch or paint the images.

Carry them with you, play with them, take them into different settings. And as you do this, explore your feelings and responses. Draw one, try and see what it means to you and if it talks in any way. Then refer to this account for interpretation, or any other that you may have or may be appropriate for you, and/or for the purpose of the consultation.

There are at least two ways you can make progress in this process. One is to contemplate a rune each day in sequential order, starting with **Feoh**, then carry it with you and explore its meanings both intuitively and educatively. The other would be to draw a random rune for each day and undertake the same examination, then see how the rune and meanings applies to that day.

From this point, you might want to follow your nose with further exploration, such as on the internet (be careful, there's a lot of rubbish there!), or to other disciplines that may contain information for you to be able to expand your appreciation. For example, as I was writing the preceding section, a series of programmes on the Viking Age came on the television, so I was able to cross-reference my writing with another viewpoint, as well as some additional information. This was synchronicity in operation, which I would see as both relevant and part of the communication process.

Divination

From this point on you will definitely need a rune set, as well as a pouch or small bag to contain them, I'd suggest. I'm also going to keep this section fairly simple with only three methods, and leave it to you to explore other permutations and combinations. One reason for this is that I want to emphasise the ground that should be covered to this point of exploration, so you do not enter into the divinatory process in a trivial manner.

At the very least, I would have expected you to explore the meanings outlined, even with my idiosyncratic approach. Such a personalised approach may encourage you to find your own meanings and interpretations, and so further the art rather than relying on rote (which, of itself, may have a personal background or slant embedded anyway). In my opinion, this is an art in progress and demands further insight and contribution, even novelty and expansion.

This is something I am actively considering, living in Australia. And, you may wonder with the apparent diversity with which the apparent rune extension appears to end, what happened with runic development under the cloak of Christianity? Well, there is a speculative 'fifth aett' that extends from the rune extension of the Futhorc, and is scattered around in the mediaeval period. So, the art and its work continues ... as we do. The *Spellbinding* section explores this area in a bit more detail.

I am fully aware there are much simpler outlines available; but the study and discipline, plus your own exploration, will stand you in good stead. If the runes haven't talked to you by now, then maybe they are not for you, and any divination process is likely to be unhelpful and – particularly if the god Loki is involved – be either inaccurate, misleading, or downright mischievous in where you may be led. Be warned.

The first method is an extension of the above familiarisation process and permits the drawing of a single rune in response to a question. The question is important and, again, should not be trivial – unless you want a trivial reply! A good question is often one that has palpable emotional significance to and for you. You may even be anxious about the answer, although these are all good signs. In general, this should be a question for which you don't have a clear response or decision in your mind already. You may want to write it out. But, at the very least, I suggest you take yourself and your runes to a setting that is significant (we will talk more about this when we come to rituals), and then speak the question out aloud.

Then close your eyes and draw a single rune from the pouch by feeling around and selecting the rune you are drawn to in a psychic way, maybe with your non-dominant hand. This rune may make itself known, or be otherwise obvious to you with a feeling or sensation in the rummaging process. Examine the rune with whatever knowledge and experience you have to date, and see how much it addresses your question and how you are affected by it. You may want to leave the space and explore the rune further in a journal (again, we'll come to this), with information from here and any other sources relevant to you.

The second method is one I routinely use in practice, if I am doing a rune reading for someone in a therapeutic context. A reading is simply that I perform the function of drawing and interpreting the runes in response to the question posed by the questioner. It is not always essential that I know what the question is to do this; in fact, and sometimes and rather obviously, it can be a hindrance to do so.

In this case, the initial stages are the same, except three runes are drawn and laid out left to right, sight unseen. The first rune represents, in literal terms, the past. In metaphoric terms, and hence of deeper significance, it is the ground, legacy, or heritage of a personal and historical nature on which you stand with respect to the question. The second is the present, or where you stand right now with respect to the question. The third is the future, or where the question and the runic responses to date are leading you; the image here is the horizon.

Past, present, and future put the sequence in a linear time framework, which I find somewhat limited. The second appreciation, with its images of what you stand upon, where you are standing right now, and what you are looking out onto, are more significant, to my way of thinking. They bring all these facets of linear time into the present rather than seeing the outcome predictively or fatalistically, offering some sort of prophetic response and interaction in the ritual process; this itself is an act of magic. The process from here is then as the first method, above.

The third method is mentioned a little hesitantly, as it is one I am still working with in terms of the extensions it can lead into that take us further afield than this commentary. The method itself is relatively straightforward. With reference to your question, draw a single rune to place in the centre of your reading space (I often use a square bandana for this setting). Then, beginning with the East and moving sunwise or deosil, draw four runes consecutively and place them in the successive compass quarters.

What I am doing here is mapping the runes – and the question – into a sacred space, a *Circle* or *Medicine Wheel*. To use this method, you will need to have some familiarity with the circle and wheel, and the attributes of the quarters. This area is not a fixed one, as these attributes can vary according to which tradition is being used, as well as variations in their significance and other associations. The medicine wheel is also deeply embedded in Tradition and culture, including the agricultural cycle and movement of the seasons (which obviously varies around the globe); notwithstanding the differing direction the sun takes in the respective hemispheres.

To do this in more detail, I have approached this method the other way around and only use it personally or with others who are familiar with the wheel. This familiarity not only comes from instruction (following a teaching approach called *Sacred Space* that I have written as an educational guide), but how this applies to rituals conducted in a sacred circle and also the ceremonies in the sweat lodge or house.

From this point start to take on a freestyle shamanic attitude and explore other methods of divination. Many commentators will give you alternatives, and you may draw from other disciplines; for example, Tarot readings have reading methods that can be applied. However, be careful about over-complicating the process. Intuitively I am also drawn to mandala-like readings, as I have a sense this is the sort of geometric patterning that the magical reality exists within and can express itself to us through, as with the third method (immediately above).

The Rune Journal

Initially, I am going to assume that you are not familiar with a diary or journal process, although I appreciate many or most readers would be. However, I will start with this assumption and lead into other possibilities from there.

In the broader context, the use of a journal has become almost indispensable in the personal growth process and is widely advocated. As the runes are used for at least this purpose, the orientation I will take for any beginner in this area will be in this wider context. If you have arrived at this point and do not use a journal, I would advise that you start one to record your experiences and outcomes with the divinatory process, at least.

The journal itself could be quite simple, like a notebook. Although giving the process a little more reverence could be facilitated by using one of those blank bound diaries that are now readily available at gift shops and newsagents. Clearly date and record your experiences, and make note of the surrounding circumstances. What drew you to asking this question? What does the reading tell you? How do you intend to apply it?

These questions inevitably lead into a wider process; the above reflections demand a context of your life, thoughts and feelings, directions and plans. This is set in a web of associations, such as partnership, family, work and friends, and the wider psychosocial context these are embedded in. In this context, a journal is a reflective tool, a place where you can express your most personal thoughts, feelings, and their consequences. I would add dreams with reflections about them, as well as any unusual experiences or happenings, such as synchronistic or 'psychic' occurrences.

Reflections on personal history are welcome, but more pertinent if initiated by circumstances and events, and always in the context of the present. Creative additions, poetic utterances, and quotes from other sources are all potentially valuable additions. This is a place where you can be most intimate with yourself, so please keep the journal safe from prying eyes; you may even protect it with a rune such as **Eolh** – **Y** – or a personal bindrune.

Many of you would already have a journal process happening, most probably with additions I have not mentioned here. But if you have not, then following the above steps will catch up with those that do, and provide a platform to further develop your own journal and the journal process. For example, as I usually get up to write early, I have a computer file that I can use as a broad journal, particularly because at this hour any dreams are more immediate and the time of day facilitates reflectiveness. I have a range of other notebooks and pads that I use as an extension of this; some are for specified purposes, particularly rune and magical work, but also notes of ideas, poetry, drawings and paintings, and the like.

The good alchemist always makes a record of his/her experiments and their outcomes. This is equivalent and your journal contains your own alchemical process, into which magical operations will be included and even direct the process.

Ritual

The journal process is a ritual; rituals were not discarded in the nursery. At times of stress and strain they emerge in often primitive and child-like form, indicating their potential place in dealing with distress, turbulence and transition, rather than being interpreted in an unhealing manner as a psychiatric problem like obsessive-compulsive disorder, or OCD. Other cultures preserve rituals in an extant form that often appeal emotionally when we visit them; we then experience their absence in our busy, preoccupied lives. We ignore them at our emotional and spiritual peril.

Reading the runes is a ritual. As with all rituals, the process itself should be in a conducive setting, maybe one sourced and set apart for this purpose, or a routine space sanctified by an act of dedication. The setting is important, as is your place in it. You may find it necessary to bathe (a ritual of purification) and dress for the occasion, even using specific clothing, such as robes, and any amulets (a protective ornament or similar). If others join you in any ritual process then it becomes more ceremonial, particularly if one of the assembled personnel conducts a ritual, with others observing or participating.

A ritual setting is sacred. The setting may have objects of reverence placed there prior to the ritual, such as swords and chalices. The elements may be represented by stone or salt (earth), water in a vessel, burning incense (fire), and a feather (air) placed in the appropriate quarters of a designated circle. A task for you is to work out which element and/or icon goes with which quarter. The circle may then be sanctified by casting it with a wand or staff, walking or circling sunwise or *deosil* from the East and back to the East again. Each quarter may then be blessed and dedicated. Then the ritual process may occur. Afterward, the process is reversed with the circle unwound *widdershins*, and the sacred space metaphorically and sometimes literally dispersed. You may appreciate the overlap and connection with the third divinatory method now.

This may all sound overwhelming if you are not familiar with rituals. However, I hope the above gives you enough information to start and experiment. Please do not neglect the imaginative process, which can augment and elaborate on the ritual structure, as well as being used at alternative times when appropriate. Imagination, in general, has a wide application in this whole domain and is the basis of any more freestyle shamanic approaches.

Of course, there is much more that could be said about ritual, as well as further instruction. This is properly a separate work, as I have created with *Sacred Space*. But I believe the above is sufficient for beginning, and I can't stress enough your own participation and experimentation. With the wonders of modern technology, you may easily search and research more, but an earlier caveat applies: Be very discerning, there is a lot of poor-quality material and instruction on the internet, and some may be downright misleading, if not potentially malicious. It will serve you well to develop your *magical muscles*, so to speak, from your own inner resources first – plus a little help from the runes and the gods.

Magic

By now you will have recognised that there is no pure stream of runic magic. The runes themselves, as seen in the introduction, are set in a wide context of history, culture, religion, mythology, and cosmology, as well as their social and psychological reflections. The magic of the runes emerges from the broad archetypal complex known as shamanism, which is a significant component in the various streams of magic that we now know of in the modern era. Some of these, such as the Kabbalah, have many different cultural and religious roots, making their compatibility difficult, if not confusing and even impossible. However, in the modern era, there is a cross-fertilisation process amongst all these Traditions, with the impetus to globalisation and the discovery of the similarity in their archetypal roots.

To this heady mix I personally add alchemy, as it was a Tradition of the ages of metal and their use. Although we now tend to see it in mediaeval form, as a process it is of great value to both magic and shamanism. Psychology is also a modern art that should not be forgotten. I am eschewing the academic, research and cognitively clinical branches here, and focusing more on the depth traditions (Jung, Reich, Hillman etc.) that work with the so-called *unconscious* – notwithstanding my earlier comment about this term – because I believe these psychologies provide a valuable link to the other Traditions and magic. Indeed, as magic is going feral with concepts such as chaos magic, and shamanism with freestyle shamanism, I believe alchemy could gain some flexibility and freedom, particularly in the healing arts. And I think that the depth psychologies are in a transitional state where a healthy injection of these other disciplines may provide much in the way of cross-fertilisation.

Indeed, I see that depth psychology is a component of what is called *Seith magic* (we will return to this topic in more detail). In its application to personal growth and development, depth psychology provides the tools of inner reflection that can help consolidate the individual self and soul, distinct from life's vicissitudes. Of course, there is a healthy mix of alchemy and shamanism in this, particularly if a therapeutic process or healing journey is undertaken, but this art can in itself be a ritual of initiation and a rite of passage.

Rune Magic

The fundamental principle here requires an act of faith: That the reality being communicated with and participated in, by the magician, is greater and more intelligent than he or she. And that magic is the process of forming an active relationship with this reality, of which we are an expression, for the purpose of being involved in the creative and evolutionary process. This bears a great responsibility and is laden with obvious pitfalls, yet the demand has been there throughout human evolution, and I would contend that is a responsibility that is not to be shirked.

Psychology, as expressed above, is the receptive arm of the process and divination is part of its expression. There is passivity in this Seith magic that is transcended as we move into the operative realms to participate co-creatively in the evolutionary journey. At one level this reality always remains mysterious and transcends even the evolution in which we are involved, yet seems to demand our involvement in the process. I will stop at this point; here we are at the borders of mysticism, and our interest is primarily in the magical process with the use of the runes in particular.

In these respects, the runes are not seen as man's invention, but as a gift of the gods. This paradoxical relationship is amplified in Odin/Woden's self-sacrifice where, pierced by a spear, he hung for nine days and nights on a great tree. In this ritual ordeal, he retrieved the runes and expressed them in eighteen charms. This poetic myth in *Havamal* is worth exploring in some detail as it contains much that we have been talking about.

However, it is not an instruction manual for the operative use of the runes, but riddles about their meaning. It was up to runemasters to interpret this material into an understanding of the runes and their application. One such attempt to match the eighteen charms to runes was made by Guido von List a little over a hundred years ago. His *Armanen runes* (or Armanen Futharkh) are a series of eighteen runes, closely based on the more magically-inclined Younger Futhark.

This is one reason why the appreciation of the runes and the process of divination are both important preliminaries, but also as an ongoing background to any operative work. I feel my appreciation of the runes is in a constant state of evolution, and that this appreciation will change and mature, even as I write this work. In this sense, we are all Odin/Woden and constantly undergoing the sacrificial process.

The essential change in operative magic is that the rune-master chooses the runes and how to use them. The issues and questions may be the same; that is, they are being used in response to some inner demand or external circumstance (including, in the shamanic sense, for another, or others). The ones used may even be selected from a divinatory type of process, rather than self-selection from your knowledge of each.

As with divination, this may be single or multiple. For example, a rune may be carved into a wooden stave or etched in a stone to be worked with in ritual, used as a *charm* (a magical act, including a *spell* or words), or maybe carried as a *talisman* (an object of magical power), *amulet* (a protective object), or otherwise sacrificed to earth, wind, water, or fire. Further runes may be used for a more comprehensive picture and here some may be bound into a combined runic form, called a bindrune. Bindrunes are often used as charms or with spells – even curses. As you can intuit here, our motives in such acts must be well examined and responsibility for any outcome recognised.

What about blood? From the remarks made in the *Introduction* blood can be viewed as an important, though not necessarily essential component. There is the symbolic significance of blood itself and therefore its metaphoric use as vitality, passion and endeavour in the process; after all, that is how it is utilised in the Christian ritual of the Eucharist. It is also inferred in the runes themselves.

Yet it is the literal aspect and use of blood that attracts considerable interest. In a world where we are distinctly phobic about it, not helped by the often-misguided modern medical attitudes toward infectious disease, manifest blood affects us deeply. It causes ambivalence; fear, yet also attraction and even excitement. To engage directly with it is profoundly emotional and is therefore a link or pathway to the spiritual. No wonder it is a significant component of rituals and obviously sacrifice, both being components of transformation.

There is a tradition that blood – your own – is used in making runes. The tools that we use shamanically and magically, such as a drum, robe, or other accoutrement, should be made by the operator. If this is not possible – say with a sword – then at the very least it should be sanctified by ritual and other processes and its 'maker' carefully chosen. For example, it is best to make your own runes; but, if you cannot, then sanctifying them with your own blood can be important to provide magical power.

Is the drawing of the blood to be done by yourself or another? It depends on the implement, the ritual, and who this other is in reference to yourself. But the common denominator is using a ritual implement, such as a knife, to cut the skin at a chosen point on the body and then to use the flowing blood in, say, colouring the shape of the rune; maybe where the shape has already been carved. The technicalities of this may require advice or assistance, and maybe it is best conducted by or assisted with by someone familiar with the territory. But make no mistake, it is a powerful and magical act.

I am going to draw a line in the sand here; it must be done somewhere after all, although we will return to sacrifice. Because, and as explained, this work is difficult to convey in this means of communication beyond a point. And for many, this point may have been reached a while ago, yet for others the desire for yet more is still present. Many of these threads will be revisited in more detail after we have examined the Futhorc itself.

The Anglo-Saxon Futhorc

Introduction

Earlier I made the comment that "from the mundane and physical levels, runic meanings can extend to the sexual, cultural, social, psychological, mythic, and spiritual". But even this could represent an incomplete list; for example, emotions, the body, as well as both physical and mental health, could be easily added. In other words, *Soulful*. It seems to me that most descriptions of runes that offer some sort of interpretation are a smorgasbord of meanings picked from some or all of these levels. The more the interpretations approach the *daily horoscope* mentality, the more they lose the depth and magic that is the essence of the runes.

I am basing this exploration on the so-called Old English Futhorc, and I will use the Bruce Dickins translation of the Old English rune poem from the transcript that George Hickes made of the original in 1705. This original was lost in a fire in 1731, so it is not known for certain whether the assignment of the poetic riddles to individual runes is entirely authentic. However, there is good agreement with the Scandinavian rune poems for the 16 common runes, so it is generally considered in academic circles that the correspondences are valid.

It should not be forgotten that the rune poem is considered to derive from a prior oral existence, originating sometime in the 8th and 9th centuries, committed to writing by Christian scribes in the 10th century, and preserved in the manuscript destroyed by the fire of 1731. The Heathen influences in the recorded script would have been considered significant, and some attempt would have been made to either edit out or otherwise modify them, following the Christianisation that proceeded in England from the early 7th century. However, at a spiritual level there is less apparent conflict between the two religious orientations, which is my feeling about the Christian influence in the poem, so there would need to be some discernment here with interpretation. Also, the rune poem describes only 29 runes, and it has already been indicated that the last four runes have spiritual connotations that may be common to both Christianity and the Heathen traditions it supposedly superseded.

If this overall assessment is considered from a historical perspective in terms of authenticity, then there would be room for argument about issues such as accuracy and validity. However, this perspective should be seen as relative, as the information we have to hand is only a very small portion of what would have been produced. In other words, and being imaginative, there would have been other variations on the shapes of runes; different assignments; other poems and riddles; and much we draw on that is mundane, uneducated, and could even be considered as graffiti.

More important to our study is the magical dimension. In reconnecting to the runic corpus, I am following a fluid and creative tradition in the company of other similar travellers. The assignments and their interpretations could be considered part of this magical process of reconnection with a spiritual tradition in a modern age, which will inevitably change and develop over time.

My emphasis from this point will be primarily psychological in the authentic sense of psyche as soul. I will focus on the physical, sexual, emotional, and intellectual aspects from the poem, and within various interpretations of runes I have read elsewhere. However, the resulting synthesis and many of the insights will be my own, with all its attendant subjectivity. The social and cultural aspects in the poem are obviously historical, so some modernisation will need to be employed on occasion.

The mythological levels are generally significant, more so in the Scandinavian material, so its relevance to English mythology – whatever that may be – is lessened; however, it is of interest from a symbolic perspective and will be referred to when this is the case. Where this causes a differing rendering of a name, as with the English Woden and Scandinavian Odin, I will offer the appropriate alternatives according to whichever rune poem is being referred to at the time.

Collectively, this psychological approach satisfies the divinatory meaning of rune usage that, as stated, I am taking from an individual or soul perspective. However, there is also a spiritual perspective embedded in all of the material, which is more apparent when the runes are employed for magical purposes. Here I suffer some of the difficulties and restrictions that would have affected early commentators, in that such an approach and the material employed is more ritualistic and conveyed best in oral tradition and its initiatory transmission. In this spiritual respect, the occult meaning of the runes as mysteries comes to the fore.

The authors I have mainly used as a background to these interpretations are Edred Thorsson, Freya Aswynn, and Jan Fries. This is a kind of cherry-picking of intellectual, intuitive, and imaginative perspectives, although the resultant synthesis is more distinctly based on my poetic appreciation of the rune poems, plus a bit of creativity – a gift from the gods! I believe this is in the spirit of the runes in our time and meets a demand, both personal and spiritual.

Runes of the Elder Futhark are set out in *aetts*, or three groups each containing eight runes. The Futhorc follows this, although the definition is less pronounced after the 24th rune. Each aett is considered to be headed and named by the first rune of the series, and to have characteristics in common with it. These features will be described at the conclusion of each aett.

I will try and use a relatively standard graphic representation of each rune, although there are variations noted by Hickes in five of them. The latter runes or extension of the Futhorc present increasing difficulties here. These variations could be considered to occur depending on the source, as well as changes over time.

This graphic representation of each rune of the Futhorc will head its further description. If the standard Elder Futhark version varies significantly, I will provide this alternative in a slightly smaller form next to the original. This is because you may have, or may only be able to obtain, the Elder Futhark version. A considered simple meaning to each rune will accompany the graphic and the preferred name in alphabetic script. Each poetic riddle or charm from the Old English rune poem will accompany the assigned rune up to the 29th. In the ensuing text, I will reference the Scandinavian rune poems where they offer a significant contrast that will inform us further, which is relatively frequently.

There will be no description of reversed or inverted runes, as this is a modern derivation – or deviation – as is the so-called blank rune (of the so-called *Self*) that provides a subtle Christianisation, already apparent enough. The various ways of using the runes takes more than sufficient account of features like reversal in a greater and more comprehensive range of meaning, which renders such descriptions simplistic, irrelevant, and even counter-productive. In short, both of these apparent additions are relatively modern and should, in my view, be discarded.

As a brief aside, both of these points are countered in the actual Futhorc itself, though not the Elder Futhark. **Calc**, the 31st rune of the Futhorc (and part of the extension beyond the Futhark) is a reversal of **Eolh**, the 15th rune. Also, **Gar,** the 33rd rune, could be considered to have functions similar to those attributed to the so-called blank rune, as will be examined later.

There is enough to do to fill in the gaps that exist, with the scant amount of information at our modern disposal, without complicating and obfuscating the overall picture with modern inaccuracies. My belief is that we start with what is extant and given, gain the wisdom of modern commentators who have explored runes from this basis, and then add a healthy dose of your own intuition and speculation – although being clear and patent about this process.

To my mind, this represents an authentic basis in which to explore the runes, modernise them, and give them a trajectory into the future. I believe this represents an active – magical – relationship with the runes and the greater forces that stand behind them, rather than imposing our own personal psychology on them, as well as the desire to make order beyond what inherently exists.

A final point before discussing the individual runes further: I am not going to describe them in neat categories directed toward meaning, be that divinatory or magical, or even – woe to you – academic. I have approached each rune in a contemplative state and written around them from my prior knowledge and understanding, infused with intuition and magical insight.

I have paid some limited attention to the phonetic and etymological aspects of the runes, where relevant; it would be a more complete work to include them, of course. Although of academic and intellectual interest, I find such approaches take me too far away from the essence and symbolic expression of the runes into modernity, as well as being a continuation of the sort of influences I am trying to both differentiate and relatively excise from the core meanings.

From the reader's – your – perspective, I would suggest that you will gain most value from my rendering by approaching each rune in this contemplative manner, read around what I have expressed, then skip to any reference to other material (such as the other rune poems) that may be mentioned and capture your interest. Then try and get a mature feeling, derived from any thoughts and emotions, of what the rune – or series of runes – means to you in the context of any question you may have posed.

In summary, and considering the Futhorc, unless stated otherwise:

- Each rune graphic is the most commonly accepted portrayal.

- The Elder Futhark alternative is given, smaller and adjacent, where it differs significantly.

- The common name of the rune is underneath, in upper case, along with the equivalent letter in Roman script, in brackets.

- The generally accepted meaning is below this, in lower case.

- There follows the relevant Old English poem for each rune (1 to 29, only).

- Other rune poems (Norse and Icelandic) are referenced in the text, if significant to the exposition.

- A summary statement of a divinatory and/or magical nature for each rune concludes the text.

- There may be a separate comment about the relationship of runes to each other, particularly the pairings in the first aett.

- There is a concluding summary of each aett.

- Other associations, such as colours, sounds, elements etc. would unnecessarily complicate and render the descriptions too much in a modern idiom; they are left for personal exploration.

And, as a kind of addendum for occult communication and ritual purposes:

- Each rune may be used as a hand gesture, or body posture (**Eolh** – ᛉ – is maybe the most obvious for these purposes).

- Some runes, but not all, will be used to illustrate these points.

- Some runes, particularly those with double vertical staves or entwining features, could be used by couples and groups, in sexual and ritual magical practice.

- It is important to see the runes not just in their individual context, but in relationship and combination with each other.

- The runes provide additional depth and significance to simple letters, due to their symbolic and metaphysical nature.

- Runes can comprise *words* and *sentences*, in a metaphoric and/or symbolic manner.

- The erotic and sexual implications of the runes are given emphasis.

Addendum on Aetts:

Each aett is named after the first letter in the sequence. This may be for convenience or magical purposes, as each aett consists of eight runes. Although the words sound similar, aett refers to a clan, not to the number. This distinction becomes less clear after rune 24 (the end of the Elder Futhark), and there will be speculation about this as we move into the extensions from rune 25 onward.

It is considered by many that the runes are divided into aettir (the plural of aett) as a kind of mnemonic device for an oral tradition, and this may well be one reason. Additionally, some commentators imply that each aett is *ruled* by a god or goddess. Whilst this may or may not be the case (as with the third aett, specifically) this might simply be a modern interpolation.

The aettir also lend themselves to a more traditional eightfold manifestation around the yearly cycle, which has ceremonial significance. There are many other permutations and combinations, which you may like to experiment with, which may have further magical significance.

So, to the first aett, that of **Feoh**:

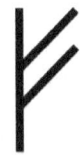

FEOH (F)

Wealth, Cattle

Wealth is a comfort to all men;
yet must everyman bestow it freely,
if he wish to gain honour in the sight of the Lord.

I would contend that *Lord* here may be a Christian addition rather than referring to a physical person, yet it accords with Heathen tradition and a physical Lord (or Lady?) as well. There is a clear indication of how wealth should be used. Both the Scandinavian poems carry a similar sentiment in using the word *discord*, as well as relating this to *kinsmen.** ** In the Norse poem this is furthered by reference to the *wolf*, which hardly needs explanation, and *forest*, usually a metaphor for what is wild and untamed. This might be a reference to the emotion that the misuse of wealth can raise.

However, the Icelandic rune poem also refers instead to wealth as *fire of the sea* and *path of the serpent*. Given the strong feminine nature of the rune, the threefold emphasis on men in the poem is an enigma, unless considered generically as reference to both men and women; alternatively, this could be another Christian influence. The contrast with the Icelandic poem is interesting, where the primal imagery is of a more feminine nature.

Cattle is historic in meaning, the original indicator and maybe arbiter of wealth in Heathen times. Wealth can be seen here as energy and the need for its circulation in the poem, otherwise it brings trouble – the discord of the other poems. In the internal sense this is personal value, a person's rank or standing; maybe another kenning of *honour in the sight of the Lord*.

The actual runic image could be of a person with arms stretched outward and upward in an act of religious supplication and receptivity. As a hand image, it resembles the version of *fuck you* with the first and second fingers in a *V* shape (although not a letter used in Anglo-Saxon times, **Feoh** sometimes fulfilled this phonetic function); so, powerful and possibly sexual, as well.

Another reference is to fire, and gold by the association to wealth. *Fire of the sea* would indicate strong emotion, even sexual energy, reinforced by the *path of the serpent* in the Icelandic poem, which recalls the kundalini energy of eastern mysticism. Mythologically gold points to Freyja, or Freo in English, goddess of the water and hence *fire of the sea*. *Tears of the sea* is a complementary phrase that a metaphor for amber, valuable as jewellery in particular, and also attributable to Freo.

A goddess of the Vanir family or race, who were often at war with the Aesir (or the race of gods, headed by Woden), Freyja/Freo also – paradoxically – taught Odin/Woden Seith, or the magic of *seething*; that is, the visionary, or sexual variety of the art. The Brisingamen necklace that adorned Freyja/Freo was obtained from the four dwarves who made it, who gave it to her in return for sexual favours with each of them on successive nights.

Feoh is rich and powerful, and refers to Freo, the goddess of fertility and sexuality. **Feoh** concerns the cultivation of feminine energies and skills, with a strong connection to fertility, magic, and witchcraft. The association of sexuality with magic is stressed. But the warning is to be generous with wealth and to involve others in any largess; maybe a feminine quality that needs to be brought to bear on what is considered a masculine undertaking in our time.

* "Wealth is a source of discord among kinsmen; the wolf lives in the forest." (Norse)

** "Source of discord among kinsmen and fire of the sea and path of the serpent." (Icelandic)

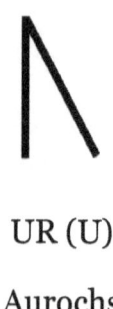

UR (U)

Aurochs

The aurochs is proud and has great horns:
it is a savage beast and fights with its horns;
a great ranger of the moors, it is a creature of mettle.

An aurochs is a primitive ox or bison now extinct, dying out early in the second millennium CE. It represents a wild, primal force, as it was unable to be tamed. Indeed, it was a challenge and initiation for young men to slay one; the gathered horns representing the trophy. The rune can then be seen as a ritual or rite of passage for men in a culture where courage and strength were highly valued. The horns, represented in the image, would be used for drinking, both socially and ritually. The runic image could also be seen as aggressive and phallic.

Ur, as a prefix, means original or primitive and refers to the core primal energy of a predominantly masculine variety. There is thus a subtle pairing of the first two runes of **Feoh** and **Ur** at this energetic masculine-feminine and erotic levels. In ways they could be seen to represent the primal forces of creation coming as they do at the beginning of all the Futharks.

By way of contrast, in the Scandinavian rune poems **Ur** rune is referred to as *lamentation of the clouds*, *snow*, and even *dross*.* ** Although often seen in a cleansing light, this meaning points to the harsh conditions of the north, as well as referring to the primal mythic and cosmological levels of the Scandinavian peoples, as these forces are a component in their creation myths.

A more tangential view is that all these associations point to **Ur** being semen, which supports the earlier phallic interpretation. This sexualised way of looking at the runes will be a feature throughout the interpretations, as the sexual components not only point to erotic mysteries, but also to the spiritual dimensions in an unbroken continuum (unlike much of Christianity). Additionally, some of these images are features of the alchemical process, which I mention here as it, too, is a feature of the runes.

A hand posture could be the thumb and fingers facing downward, with a natural space between. This is very prehensile, and reinforces the primal power of the rune. Without sounding sexist, it also implies masculinity (in both men and women). The overall impression is of contained or inherent power. No wonder this beast represented an initiatory challenge to young men at many levels. In the OE poem above, *Mettle* indicates a controlled use of power, and the double reference to *horn* reinforces this, as well as its indirect and colloquial sexual implications.

Ur is raw primal energy and vitality; it is the wild side of our nature that is untamed. Yet it is also the basis of our consciousness through our instinctual nature, here seen in a powerful and creative light. Referred to as shadow, unconscious, or other pejorative terms, it could also relate to the *Underworld* that underpins the daily world and within which the primal and instinctual forces reside. Think dwarves (who, as smiths and metalworkers, are proto-alchemical), or Grendel and his mother in the Beowulf saga.

* "Dross comes from bad iron; the reindeer often races over the frozen snow." (Norse)

** "Lamentation of the clouds and ruin of the hay-harvest and abomination of the shepherd." (Icelandic)

Pairing: That both **Feoh** and **Ur** relate to beasts, domestic and wild, is itself of interest. And that these two runes should be at the very beginning of all the Futharks may be no accident. The cow, Audhumla, featured early in the cosmological myth after fire and ice came together and started the creation process. The phrase *sight of the lord* in **Feoh** would be an interesting one if the *he* referred to *she* instead.

In the modern revivalism of witchcraft, called Wicca, the primal pairing is the lord and lady. The lord in Wicca is a horned god, as is the aurochs, indicating another association to this primal pairing. In mythic lore Freo's partner (or brother) is Frey, a Vanic god. It may be stretching the association to see Frey associated with the **Ur** rune, but it makes for interesting speculation.

There are also some primal alchemical features in these two runes that are tantalising with what is to emerge later. This dualistic pairing frequently weaves its way down the first series or aett of the Futhorc, as will be seen with the runes that follow, and continues suggestively throughout.

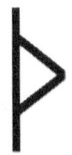

THORN (Th)

Giant, Thorn

The thorn is exceedingly sharp,
an evil for any knight to touch,
uncommonly severe on all who sit among them.

In Germanic cosmology, the giants preceded the gods and man, yet remain as part of the world. The giants represent the forces of chaos, and it is Thor (OE Thunor, or *thunder*) who keeps them under control. In psychological terms the giants represent the subconscious; those forces at the borderline of awareness that we need to keep in check. It is interesting that it is Thor who does this, because although he is a god, he has many of the giants' features.

This controlling power Thor is represented by his hammer, often worn as an amulet against the dominance of these primal forces or, more pertinently, as the symbolic force used to deal with them. This is a distinct contrast to the use of the Christian cross in protection from evil, although with a little imagination the cross could become Thor's hammer!

The Scandinavian rune poems recognise the giants to be a danger to women, presumably because of their voracious sexual appetites.* ** The Norse poem accentuates chaos as *misfortune*. In this connection, in character the giant is not unlike an incubus, considered evil by the Church. Maybe it is this demonic side of the rune that threatens the establishment order and why, apart from the reference to *evil thing*, the rune is edited severely and changed to a plant in the Futhorc. I would further question whether the *evil thing for any knight to touch* may also have later Christian as well as misogynistic overtones; as well as a euphemism for 'women' and their inherent sexual nature perhaps?

Although harsh and somewhat severe, the Old English rune poem carries less of the severity of the other poems, or their inherent meaning within the Futharks. There is an unfortunate and progressive demythologisation of the runes from this point in the Futhorc, and **Thorn** marks the tone. This can be seen in the image, where the primal association with thunder becomes the thorn of a plant, readily seen in the shape of the rune.

Although there are similarities of domain here with **Ur**, being the Underworld or unconscious, there is one significant difference; **Thorn** has a more aggressive, violent, and has a warlike quality. This is reinforced by his hammer, which may resemble that of the smith and hence alchemy, but is frequently seen in the myths as violent and destructive. Uncomfortable though it may be, this all touches on the role of these forces in our lives, which are poorly integrated in the modern era. The demythologisation of **Thorn** in the Futhorc does not mitigate the issue; it simply hides it.

It may be with the magical overtones here that thorns can be a hedge, which mark a boundary between civilisation and the wild, providing a symbolic similarity between the differing runic systems. But it is one that can be crossed over, hence the fear of giants amongst women, and the implication in other texts that the magician is often a *fence-sitter* (in Druidry he or she is known as a *hedge-druid*). The magician is thus capable of travelling into territory that others would not dare to enter.

Thorn is at the borderline of human consciousness and represents the fears of the instinctual and primal emotional forces that stand in the realms apparently beyond the human, but can impact upon it. Yet this balance is maintained by one almost of their own, Thor, or else by a magician. It requires one who moves between the worlds with familiarity to provide a balance. Despite all of this, **Thorn** is considered a dangerous rune, used with care, and is often utilised in spells and curses.

* "Giant causes anguish to women; misfortune makes few men cheerful." (Norse)

** "Torture of women and cliff-dweller and husband of a giantess." (Icelandic)

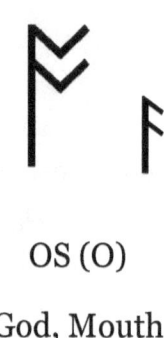

OS (O)

God, Mouth

*The mouth is the source of all language,
a pillar of wisdom and a comfort to wise men,
a blessing and joy to every knight.*

This is one of 4 runes in the Old English Futhorc that differ from those in the 24 rune Germanic or Elder Futhark. In the Futhark this rune loses the two up-stokes that come from the stave. Unlike the remaining 3 alternative runes, this rune in the Futhark has a different phonetic attribute of 'A' and is found in the rune extension as rune 26 **Aesc**, to which we will come. This differentiation process may indicate one of the ways the Futhorc has 'evolved' from the Elder Futhark.

As a brief aside, the misogynistic trend in the rune poem continues, and further indicates the influence of Christianity throughout the entire poetic corpus. By contrast the Icelandic poem exemplifies ON Odin, or Woden in OE, in his threefold and hence magical form.* (nb: ON = Old Norse, OE = Old English)

In fact, it is difficult to read this stanza of the rune poem without its Christian influence. The Icelandic poem talks of the God as Allfather (a common title for Odin/Woden), prince of Asgard (the dwelling of the Aesir gods), and lord of Valhalla (where warriors killed in battle go to, a kind of heathen heaven). Maybe it was this association that conflicted with the Christian perspective. However, by contrast the Norse poem refers to an estuary, the *mouth* of a river, and a scabbard; the repository of the sword that is often synonymous with the soul of the warrior (see the rune **Rad** that follows).**

Yet the runic influence of Odin/Woden remains, as earlier referred to, in his capacity as the god of poetry and Galdor. Galdor refers to runic and poetic magic, the province of Odin/Woden and the complement of Seidr/Seith, the witchcraft of the Vanir goddess Freyja/Freo. Both poetry and rune magic employ language – words – and I have earlier referred to the association of the word with the divine.

The image itself in the Old English poem reinforces the mouth, when the horizontal strokes are seen as lips in the act of speaking. This is an interesting development in the Futhorc, because in the Elder Futhark this rune is called **Ansuz,** is represented by the letter *A* and is called God; specifically the god Odin, who practised Galdor magic based on the word and poetry. As with the preceding rune **Thorn** there is a demythologisation process apparent with the development of the Futhorc from the Elder Futhark.

It should be remembered that, beyond the Christian influence in any of these changes, we are dealing with an oral culture. The word was considered powerful, and the retention of words in memory was a vital and trained function, as exemplified by Celtic Druidry in its extensive training, considered to be nineteen years. The lack of commitment to writing is sometimes seen as primitive, but if we get beyond this prejudice, we can start to unravel lost wisdom. Words form the basis of Galdor magic, and are an inherent part of poetry, charms and spells, as well as with their use in ritual and magical operations more generally.

Yet all these rather mixed ambiguities are overcome when we see this rune to relate to consciousness (*pillar of wisdom*) and to have moved beyond the borderline image of the **Thorn** rune. In this respect, **Os** represents the end of the evolution of the primal forces through the giants into the gods ... next we will come to man.

Os represents the divine within us, or the transcendent self. Our innate ability to use words and verbalise them in a more poetically-inclined manner indicates our continued relationship with our own divinity, beyond their simple use as a means of communication. Yet **Os** is more than this; it represents our relationship to our own innate wisdom and the ability to express and manifest it in speech, as well as to use it for magical purposes.

* "Aged Gautr and prince of Ásgardr and lord of Vallhalla." (Icelandic)

** "Estuary is the way of most journeys; but a scabbard is of swords." (Norse)

Pairing: Both the **Thorn** and **Os** runes overtly display a more transpersonal, mythic and cosmological quality that is not as evident in **Feoh** and **Ur**. It is as if they stand behind and beyond our human existence and the primal forces of creation, yet reinforce and influence it significantly. However, they do retain a connection, if themes like sexuality, power and magic are examined more closely. In the threefold system of the shamanically-inclined Heathen – underworld, middle world, and overworld – and its extension to the more differentiated and complex nine worlds of the Norse, these runes are a reminder of the forces that stand beyond yet impact upon our middle world, Midgard, or Midyard. Yet, even with the demythologisation the image of the gods looms large in this pair. There is an impression of power and its management in the shamanic image of Woden, to whom we will return.

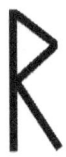

RAD (R)

Riding, Road

*Riding seems easy to every warrior while he is indoors
and very courageous to him who traverses the high-roads
on the back of a stout horse.*

At the mundane level the meaning of **Rad** seems obvious; it encapsulates riding, the rider, the riding vehicle (the horse) and the road. But in the poem it is not the physical structure of the road that is being represented, it is the road as journey, demanding physical enactment. It is about the process of riding rather than the structure of the road itself.

The image portrays a movement to the right, like someone walking, and is relatively easy to represent physically. It would be difficult to represent with one hand, as was suggested with **Feoh**, but is possible using the first three fingers in profile; give it a try. It may help here to think of the silhouette images produced by using the hands between a light source and a screen. Though maybe inexact, these sorts of alternatives are possible to those well-practiced, and easily lend themselves to subtle forms of communication not noticed by a casual observer and hence available for a secret nature; after all, that is what the runes are, by name (secret, whisper) and magical usage.

The significance of the horse is important; it even occupies a special place with the 19th rune **Eh** (horse), which is paired with the 20th rune **Man** (man) in the Futhorc. The relationship between a man (a warrior in the poem) and his horse is important, although in the poem the horse is – needs to be – stout. The Scandinavian rune poems reinforce the stress involved, with riding being *the worst thing for horses* and *toil of the steed* in the Norse and Icelandic poems respectively.* **

Yet there is more implied here. The journey is not just physical, it is also spiritual. Woden rides a great eight-legged steed across the sky, Sleipnir, reinforcing this connection. The difference is that Woden journeys between the worlds, rather than a linear journey in physical reality. This might explain the reference to the *finest sword* in the Norse poem, which is an extension of the comments made in the earlier rune **Os**. For the warrior, the sword is synonymous with or the repository of his soul, and the journey would therefore be between the worlds, and ultimately to Valhalla at the completion of his time on earth … preferably killed in battle.

Recalling the comments about **Thorn**, there is a further reflection here of the warrior culture, war, power as strength, and violence. This is mentioned to reinforce not only the presence of these forces in an ongoing manner in these earlier societies, but also to note the lack of direct relationship that we have with them in the 21st century. It is as if because we are not embracing war and violence, we are also not addressing the spiritual aspects of it that were present in these societies, to our collective detriment. Violence, death, eros, and the sacred are profoundly related. Maybe the role that the martial arts can play here in our era should be heeded.

After the more transpersonal images and meanings within the preceding two runes, and their derivation from the primal opposites that creates both them (gods and giants, among other beings) and we humans, the runes have returned to a more personal theme with the image of a journey. Such a journey requires a *stout horse* that may be, literally, the body in physical reality. But beyond this, the horse may be – like Woden's – the vehicle that contains all our consciousness rests upon, being the soul.

With the association to Woden this rune indicates the Galdor aspect of magic, as the features of this rune are inherently masculine. Although **Rad** also extends to Seith magic and ecstasy, much as Woden did in his own development, which will be more apparent as we move next to the **Cen** rune. Like a lot of runes there are also some hidden or occult sexual implications as well.

In all these respects, the **Rad** rune can be seen as shamanistic and the horse could be seen as a 'power animal'. The rune is about the journey of the soul and the inclusion of the physical body in this process, by whatever mystic-magical process the aspirant chooses. In the modern spiritual context, it represents the wisdom that the journey is more important than the destination.

* "Riding is said to be the worst thing for horses; Reginn forged the finest sword."

** "Joy of the horsemen and speedy journey and toil of the steed."

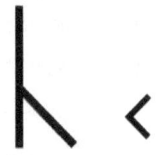

CEN (C)

Torch, Light

The torch is known to every man by its pale, bright flame;
it always burns where princes sit within.

Cen is relatively easily represented, by the body and the hands. It is also a hard C like a *K*, which it actually is in the Futhark, although in certain Old English words it is like a *Ch* sound. This overlap between these two Roman letters continues even today, although it is not isolated to **Cen**. The vowels, in particular, are often difficult to nail down with simple correspondences, not only between the Old English and Roman scripts, but also between the various Futharks.

Rather like the **Ur** rune, when compared to the other rune poems, **Cen** apparently demonstrates two clear meanings; here that is of a torch, yet in the other Scandinavian poems it is an ulcer or sore. However, this divergence diminishes significantly when the more metaphorical and sacred levels of interpretation are explored.

The connecting point between the two is the focus on death with *death makes a corpse pale* (Norse), and *abode of mortification* (Icelandic), both following the common phrase *fatal to children.**
** The reference to death in the Old English rune poem is hinted at by *pale, bright flame*. The focus in the Scandinavian rune poems may talk of the loss of children with the harshness of the times,

death at birth or in infancy, dietary deprivation, and disease; although the Futhorc poem extends this to burning and where *princes sit within* (if there is a clear connection between the various poems). Again, at the obvious level this may refer to the torch and burning as cremation, but does it refer to more, as with the burning of a sore or ulcer, or the fever of infectious disease? Further, is *prince* symbolic of inner richness and *within* a reference to inner, spiritual development?

It is here that we step into the shamanic level of kenning (itself a word based on **Cen**). In this framework wounding, disease and death are seen as steps of transformation facilitated by the *inner fire*. This reminds us of kundalini, even sexual energy, or the catalytic process of change in alchemy. It is my understanding that this is the core complex that **Cen** represents.

Added to this perception is that there may be a direct sexual component in **Cen**, and that the images may refer to the core of sexuality within the woman; the kundalini reference above reinforces this. That this is ambiguously nominated as a torch or a wound further compounds the enigma. It seems deeply mysterious, reinforced by the association of **Cen** with the Anglo-Saxon derived word, *cunt*.

There are also three manifestations of this rune as an image across the Futharks: the **Cen** of the Futhorc as described; the Younger Futhark **Kaun** rendered with the angular stave moving upward and outwards to the right, as a mirror of **Cen** around the horizontal plane, and the Elder Futhark **Kenaz** where these two angular staves join as a *C* with a 90-degree juncture and without the vertical stave. This degree of variation is unique, and adds to the enigmatic nature of this rune. Also, if each of the rune graphics is looked at, they can all be seen to be 'incomplete' in a pictographic and maybe symbolic way when compared to other similar runes. To my mind, this reinforces the wounding and trauma interpretation.

I find this the most mysterious of runes; **Cen** indicates the complexity and inherent symbolic wisdom in the Futharks, unlike most, if not all the others. Although beyond our capacity here, this rune has sufficient inherent information for a wide and deep level of exploration that could then reveal a methodology and wisdom for all the runes, even if it involves some filling in of gaps with intuitive guesswork.

Cen is a rune of shamanic significance, because of its association with wounding, death, and even enlightenment as the torch, if not simply a light for the journey (**Rad**). It has powerful, deep, and enigmatic feminine associations that include sexuality, but appear to extend to spiritual mysteries beyond. **Cen** represents the feminine as a path to spiritual realisation, which includes authentic sexuality as a tool. It manifests and radiates Seith magic. The darker aspects may be more relative when this rune is considered in association with others.

* "Ulcer is fatal to children; death makes a corpse pale." (Norse)

** "Disease fatal to children and painful spot and abode of mortification." (Icelandic)

Pairing: **Rad** and **Cen** form a complementary and shamanic pair. As with all these pairings of the first aett it is of value to read them together to gain some of the subtleties of meaning that each contains within the other (rather like Yin and Yang).

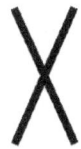

GYFU (G)

Gift

*Generosity brings credit and honour, which support one's dignity;
it furnishes help and subsistence
to all broken men who are devoid of all else.*

There are no correspondences to this rune poem in the Scandinavian rune poems; it is one of the eight runes that are dropped from the Elder in the composition of the Younger Futhark. Some of the wisdom of this reduction can be seen in the poem itself, where there are some inherent similarities to **Feoh** and **Cen**.

From the word associations in the various Germanic tongues, this rune is seen as a representing a gift. In the social sense, and reinforced in **Feoh**, this can be seen as the gift of generosity and its reciprocation. At a somewhat deeper level of meaning, it can relate to the giving and taking of relationship, and hence its common symbolic application to love and marriage, as indicated in the rune image itself. **Gyfu** is therefore commonly used as a rune in a bindrune complex.

Interestingly, the symbol X is used as a negation (wrong answers, for example) and XXX is a modern symbol for explicit sexual content, such as pornography. It also, and commonly, represents a kiss. There is a lot of ambiguity here, some of which may relate to Christianisation (interestingly, Christ can be represented as *X*) and the concept of taboo. My impression is there is a lot of sexual mystery to this rune.

The image lends itself to various forms of physical representation, from the open and vulnerable spread-eagle, crossed arms, sexual union, and cross-fingers; although the last could also apply to the rune, **Nyd**, which I favour.

The *broken man* brings us back to shamanism. In **Gyfu** the gift of generosity is that of the gods, or spiritual world, to mankind. It can then be seen as a rune of wounding and healing, and reinforces the shamanic theme that runs through all the Futharks. The wounding of the broken man can be physical, but even in modern parlance it may imply a breakdown in the mental realms. This is one of the profound tenets of shamanism, and paints a different picture of where the modern notion of a *mental breakdown* may lead, and how it can be dealt with in a healing manner by the *generosity* of the gods; that is, that the spiritual world is the one that ultimately heals mental distress.

The converse notion of gift is of sacrifice. Here there is a subtle appreciation that any gift of healing, essentially from the gods, implies a sacrifice on the recipient's part. Hence the reason for the cooperative relationship with the spiritual world and the sacrifice we give – maybe only in token or symbolic form – in ritual and ceremony. Indeed, Odin/Woden's sacrifice of himself led to the discovery of the runes for mankind. The self-sacrifice of Jesus should not be forgotten in this light.

By its very nature, **Gyfu** is erotic and generous. The giving and receiving has many levels of kenning, including the sexual. It is essentially a rune of healing, be this sexual, emotional distress, or mental turmoil. It indicates that openness and vulnerability to the other – be this a person or the divine – are important components of health and healing.

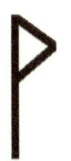

WYN or WYNN (W)

Joy, Pleasure

Bliss he enjoys who knows not suffering, sorrow nor anxiety, and has prosperity and happiness and a good enough house.

Wyn, sometimes **Wynn**, also has no Scandinavian rune poem correspondence and seems relatively obscure. The rune shape seems an upward progression of **Thorn** and has a somewhat humanised appearance if looked at in differing ways. Interestingly, these are two runes that persisted in the English language and were included in the Roman alphabet in their runic form for some centuries after it was adopted, in preference to others of the Futhorc. Their contrasting nature is intriguing and maybe reconciled with **Wyn** being a progression or consciousness of the more primal forces of **Thorn**, or it may imply a deeper unity.

The word itself also lends itself to a sexual interpretation with the literal interpretation of *winning* and *winsome*. There are some distinct similarities to the preceding (and maybe paired) **Gyfu**, which makes me wonder about both their inclusion here, and their absence in the 16 rune Younger Futhark (as represented by the Norse and Icelandic rune poems). They are lighter, playful, even erotic.

This sexual aspect underlies the idea of ecstasy and leads to the shamanic dimension, almost by definition, as the shaman is considered the master of the art of ecstasy. In this respect, the god who may be associated with **Wyn** is Woden, and even the runic name has a certain similarity. Of further interest is that **Wyn** has the same root as the Latin Venus (the goddess of love) and the race of the Vanir, of whom the goddess Freo is a member, with all her sexual and pleasurable connections.

You may recall that it was Freo who taught Woden Seith, or magic that includes the sexual or tantric variety. All these connections are tantalising, as well as giving a distinctly different flavour to much that has been encountered so far in the rune poems. Sexual magic is inferred here, with both the power implications, and also reference to the will; this shines a different light on sado-masochism, possibly?

The shamanic element is reinforced by the first line of the poem, where bliss (or ecstasy) could be seen as the transformation of *suffering, sorrow* and *anxiety*, rather than its exclusion: Suffering is the more mental aspect of pain, as sorrow is of grief, and anxiety is in a direct manner. So, we are dealing here with the more mental and spiritual aspects of existence, although a *good enough house* could refer to the body. I suspect it implies a balance of wealth and prosperity, as implied elsewhere in the runes.

Wyn may also refer to the aspect of Woden that is most magical; that is, the exercise of the *will*. In magical and shamanic terms, the employment of the will is seen as essential. In our modern era, the will is often equated with the term ego and the latter given a somewhat deprecatory view. This is unfortunate, and where psychology can be a tool of an establishment that would disempower the individual, as the correct use of the will is essential to personal growth and transformation, which is the very essence of magic. I would add to this that the will, particularly in the magical realms, necessitates an awareness and conscious integration of power; something shamanism appreciates.

Pairing: **Gyfu** and **Wyn** form a pair that have similarities, rather than some of the contrasts of the earlier pairings. They also provide a lightness and an optimism that is often lacking in the preceding runes, as well as having a more distinct sexual, magical, and shamanic flavour. It is possible that these runes are the basis of sexual magic and practice. I am amused by the letter W being a *double* U and the implications of this.

The **Feoh** aett: There is an implied pairing of the runes in dyads, as well as a more mythic progression through the aett, such that the **Feoh** aett could be seen as outlining a creation mythology of the northern peoples, as well as an evolution and progression of the shamanic and magical influences. If this is true, we may well see that each aett tells a different story, although I would expect the magical input to be a continuous theme; after all, this is the prime intent, purpose and meaning of the runes!

Now to the second aett, that of **Hagal**:

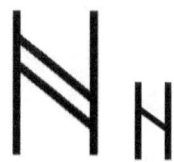

HAGAL or HAEGL (H)

Hail

Hail is the whitest of grain;
it is whirled from the vault of heaven
and is tossed about by gusts of wind
and then it melts into water.

It may be that the differences in the names represents one between the literal and metaphoric use of this rune; because **Haegl** may mean hail, but **Hagal** could also refer to a downfall or catastrophe. The rune implies this with the middle bars moving down between the two vertical staves. (An alternative shape for **Hagal** in the Anglo-Saxon tradition has only one bar, like in the Futhark, and is often used interchangeably.) These variations may also express the process of transition of this and other runes from the Elder Futhark to the Futhorc.

There are some similarities to the **Ur** rune here, which reflects the primal ice of creation and indicates a creative function to **Hagal**, in spite of its rather ominous and obvious interpretation. In these respects, **Hagal** also represents winter.

The creative function is indicated in the fact that all three rune poems refer to hail as grain, either as whitest or cold/coldest (Scandinavian rune poems). In the Old English poem, there seems to be quite a longish description of this changing process, although the connection here with *heaven* is of spiritual interest, inferring that even in the darkness of winter (and the most severe catastrophe) there is a spiritual and shamanic component in operation. There is also an implied relationship to the seasons and the agricultural cycle here.

Other rune rows often have a more clearly pictographic representation of hail as a six-sided star shape, like a snowflake as with **Ior** in the rune extension of the Futhorc. The Old Norse poem refers to *Christ created the world of old*, which may refer to the creative and mythological aspect of hail, and *Christ* being a later interpolation, or maybe in exchange for Odin/Woden?* In the Icelandic poem, the reference to hail as *sickness of serpents* is enigmatic.** I suspect a deep association between **Hagal** and **Ior**.

Serpents appear on more than one occasion in the poems; it is tempting to read this phrase in either a shamanic or tantric manner: or even both. Certainly, the image suggests tantra with two figures conjoined. As reference to animals is not common in the Futharks, so this may be significant, particularly because the serpent may have further mythological associations, as in *worm* or *dragon*. And here in **Hagal** are the serpents entwined, coupling? Is this a northern caduceus, which also has a single snake or double snake representation?

Hagal indicates that even in the worst adversity there is a creative potential that is spiritually inspired, and to stick it out. It could refer to deep primal feeling states that are not readily available emotionally. This could be the sort of counsel given to someone with severe depression and engaged with creatively, rather than taking recourse to drugs to alleviate the suffering, which would only further block the creative and transformative process. **Hagal** reminds us that a full life is not a bed of roses or permanent state of happiness.

* "Hail is the coldest of grain; Christ created the world of old." (Norse)

** "Cold grain and shower of sleet and sickness of serpents." (Icelandic)

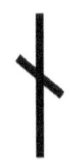

NYD (N)

Need, Necessity

Trouble is oppressive to the heart;
yet often it proves a source of help
and salvation to the children of men,
to everyone who heeds it betimes.

An alternative name for **Nyd** is *constraint*, which the image implies with the crossing stave as a limit or blockage to the central stave. An alternative image is of two fire sticks, where the repeated friction of rubbing together ultimately leads to a fire. The term *need-fire* is derived from this and sees conflict also as transition, as the need-fire was used for initiation rituals with the participant leaping through it. A literal view is to see the image as the crossed-fingers as a charm for good luck.

In contrast, the Scandinavian poems emphasise the constraint and oppressive aspects without the liberating aspect of the Old English poem.* ** By now, this would seem a feature of the runes generally and makes me ask questions about the function and purpose of the Scandinavian poems: Maybe the Christian influence is stronger than has been given credit and has transcribed them in a more negative and repressive manner, thus – hopefully – alienating them from the populace. These poems are of later origin than the runes themselves, being composed in the Christian era of both nations.

Nyd can also mean a knot, and here the Norns, or the three weavers of fate, can be seen as a possible association. **Nyd** is thus closely related with the enigmatic northern concept of *'wyrd'*, for which I like this quote:

"Wyrd (or sometimes Weird) is a term for concepts roughly corresponding to those of fate or destiny but involving complex interactions of universal necessity and individual choice within a cosmos beyond any fixed notions or concepts of mortal minds."

The use of the word 'necessity' links wyrd back to the image of **Nyd**.

In the poem and reflecting on wyrd, *betimes* may refer to the future, and hence taking on *trouble* as a transition to *salvation*. In other words, if we avoid trouble *to the heart*, we may also miss a richer future. Through the veils of Christian influence lies a deeper aspect to suffering and trauma that is more shamanic in tone. Correctly, this restores *trouble* to the individual and their life quest, rather than displacing it onto another.

The focus on the heart is interesting. Whilst we moderns may relate it to emotion and feeling, during these times it was often considered as the centre of the personality, somewhat similarly to how we now see the brain. Does this represent a shift in how we see embodied consciousness? And I am not implying here that such a shift necessarily represents progress or evolution; in fact, I don't think it does. Or does it imply that the Heathen Mentality saw feelings as superior in the psychic economy, and more related to their more immanent relationship to the Soul?

Here with **Nyd**, as elsewhere throughout the Futhorc, the guidance in how to deal creatively, purposefully, and shamanically with mental turmoil is readily apparent. There are hints to take a leap into the unknown. There is an accent in the runes – and hence in the times – of turmoil, trouble, and conflict, but the overwhelming attitude is one of acceptance of these forces as factors in our fate and personal evolution. This reinforces the concept of wyrd, or destiny, which is a profound influence for northern peoples and present particularly in **Nyd**.

* "Constraint gives scant choice; a naked man is chilled by the frost. (Norse)

** "Grief of the bond-maid and state of oppression and toilsome work. (Icelandic)

I

IS (I)

Ice

Ice is very cold and immeasurably slippery;
it glistens as clear as glass and most like to gems;
it is a floor wrought by the frost, fair to look upon.

The image here, somewhat like an icicle, is self-evident. The poem describes some of the dangers (*cold, slippery*), qualities (*wrought by frost*), and also some of the beauty (*gems, fair to look upon*) that is inherent in the danger. The choice of the word *immeasurably* is intriguing as it means beyond measurement, something infinite. This all indicates the strange and paradoxical attraction that danger may hold for us, and represented by **Is**.

The floor is something to be crossed, and the Norse poem refers to it as a *broad bridge*.* The poem goes on to say that *the blind man must be led*, indicating that crossing is a necessity or fate requiring assistance, because the *blind man* cannot see or may be unable to see this passage. But with the *blind man*, who or what does the leading? Although tangential, the bridge that connects the everyday world, Midgard, with Asgard (the realm of the gods) is called *bifrost*, which may be translated as "the shaking or trembling rainbow". There is no direct literal connection here with the *wrought by the frost* mentioned above, or the frequent references to frost in the poems, because bifrost is a firey bridge! Yet I still find the association interesting: Fire and Ice are the two primal elements of creation in Norse mythology, after all!

In a psychological sense, ice can be enchanting and cause us to become stuck; there is frequent mythological reference to this state, as well as in fairy stories, particularly if involving the Ice or Snow Queen. The Icelandic poem even refers to the *destruction of the doomed.*** Doom being a more sinister aspect of fate, or wyrd, and more like the term *fatal*. It is as if we must beware of becoming entranced, or fixed, by forces that seem beautiful and enchanting. It is also that we may need other forces to lead us (as a blinded or *blind man*) from this state; a hint of a deeper spiritual reality as exemplified by bifrost and the Norse rune poem.

Is is a challenging rune. In isolation, it is a place of stasis with impending challenges, both fearful and attractive. Beyond this, it is a deeply ambivalent rune. Ice is one of the primal components of the creation myth, so maybe the ambivalence reflects – rather like Yin and Yang – the essential interconnectedness of what seem irreconcilable opposites. In this respect, **Is** represents very deep feeling states beyond emotionality, that demand to be worked with, a little like the fire of creation or the alchemical furnace. This fire could be that of deep emotion, such as desire, passion, or sexuality that thaws Ice and reveals what is hidden and static within us.

Is is a rune of depth and not to be taken lightly or dealt with trivially. **Is** invites us to be still in the face of impending challenges and to allow the deeper forces at work to emerge into clarity, either with passive attention or more active magical intent, to direct us through what obstructs us.

* "Ice we call the broad bridge; the blind man must be led." (Norse)

** "Bark of rivers and roof of the wave and destruction of the doomed." (Icelandic)

The first three runes: Unlike the first aett, where we looked at the runes as four sets of binaries, or pairs, the first three runes of the second aett could be looked at together. The references and associations to fate, wyrd, and doom in **Is** recalls the comments around **Nyd**. If **Nyd** represents one of the Norns (the female weavers of fate) and the future, then **Is** would represent the Norn of the present. Then where is the Norn of the past? The closest association may well be **Hagal** and, if so, these three runes can be seen to form a functional unity, which they seem to be in both image and tone. Additionally, the order past, future, present is at variance to our linear concept of time of being past – present – future, which itself is worthy of contemplation.

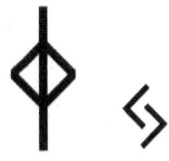

GER (Y)

Year, Harvest

*Summer is a joy to men, when God, the holy King of heaven,
suffers the earth to bring forth shining fruits
for rich and poor alike.*

The association with the year appears present in the central part of the image, and **Ger** represents the whole year, even though the poem calls it summer. In the Elder Futhark this central image, minus the stave, is split lengthways and separated a little vertically, so that it looks like a **Kenaz** rune with its mirror-image circling each other. The year divided into two halves of summer and winter is more distinctly recognised in the north, both in the ritual cycle, as well as in the more pronounced daily changes that occur progressively towards the north pole.

In the north, the year began with the beginning of winter rather than in mid-winter, at Samhain or Halloween. Traditionally also, the dusk or night marks the beginning of the next day. These different emphases bear reflection with their spiritual significance around dark and lightness. Summer is the culmination of the year and its bountifulness, with the continuing theme of spiritual balance and equality – *rich and poor alike*. The emphasis here is strongly on the agricultural cycle and its variations.

Both the Scandinavian poems use the word *boon* here, and neither have the seemingly strong Christian message, which stands in paradoxical contrast to my comments in the earlier **Nyd** rune.* ** However, this may all simply represent the mixing of cultures and ideologies over place and time, as there are many such paradoxes in the rune material we have to hand. In this particular rune the Christian message is loud and clear, even to the use of the word *suffers*. It may be that *God, the holy King of heaven* replaces a Heathen identity here.

Interestingly, in the Norse poem *Frodi* is mentioned. Although this name could refer to a Danish king (and add a little further enigma to the *King* reference in the Old English poem), the name is possibly an eponym for the god Freyr. In Norse mythology, Freyr is the ruler of peace, fertility and sunshine, and is the son of the sea god Njörd. Both Freyr and Freyja/Freo are of the Vanir race, and as gods they hark back to a more agricultural time, prior to the popular image of northern people in the Viking era.

The repeated inclusion of these figures in the rune series (Freyja/Freo in particular), as well as their incorporation into the pantheon of the northern gods indicates that progression of a culture can also be by incorporation, rather than domination and exclusion, as is too often the case with Christianity.

The letter Y represents **Ger** rather than G, which is found in **Gyfu**. In other German languages it became a J, which did not enter the English language until many centuries later. Hence the sound of the word *year*. Phonetically, this rune is connected in the Younger Futhark by **Ar** to **Ass/Os** and hence the god Woden, who may be the god that the *holy King of heaven* has replaced in the Old English poem. This pattern of interpolation will be readily apparent now.

Ger is the twelfth rune, marking the turning point in the 24-rune Elder Futhark. It represents plenty, as well as our profound connection to the earth we live on and (indirectly) to our bodies and the welfare of both, which are ultimately deeply connected. It represents both general bountifulness and ritual thanksgiving to the blessings of life and well-being. The mandala shape of **Ger** indicates balance and wholeness, but of a fluid and dynamic nature.

* "Plenty is a boon to men; I say that Frodi was generous." (Norse)

** "Boon to men and good summer and thriving crops." (Icelandic)

EOH (EO)

Yew (tree)

The yew is a tree with a rough bark,
hard and fast in the earth, supported by its roots,
a guardian of flame and a joy upon an estate.

Here – and in the next two runes – the Old English rune poem has no Scandinavian equivalent in this position of the Futhorc, yet it does appear as the final rune of the Younger Futhark as **Yr** (combining **Eoh** with **Eolh**, the 15th rune), using a shape that is an inverted **Eolh**.

These manipulations reflect much of the evolving phonetics of each language, particularly the vowels, which can be an additional point of potential confusion that I am attempting to minimise here. The letter *Y* is close to *EO*, which has been nominated here, but is by no means certain. As with **Ger**, the connection between the consonants and vowels here are not as clear and orderly as we might believe or like them to be.

We will also come across the yew again, but there is a differentiation in the Futhorc between the tree yew, as here in **Eoh**, and its common usage as a bow, which is also called **Yr** in the rune extension of the Futhorc. By contrast, in the Scandinavian rune poems the two aspects stand side-by-side within the **Yr** rune; I include them here even though they are not strictly associated with **Eoh**, because of their relevance, as well as because these poems would not otherwise be mentioned in this part of the study.* ** However, it can be seen that whilst the Norse poem is relevant to **Eoh** here, the Icelandic poem is more applicable to its namesake **Yr** in the rune extension.

The associations with the yew tree in northern cultures are invariably and maybe paradoxically life-embracing, making their connection with graveyards and hence with death itself of interest. This may be reflected in Churches being built on existing sacred areas of the Heathen peoples they supervened, whose attitude to death was by no means as pessimistic as the Christian worldview, thus effecting a further level of psychological and social control. The Heathen had a very different appreciation of death, it may be recalled.

The yew is the oldest and strongest of trees, and can live up to 2000 years. Its strength is one reason it is used for the making of bows, as well as being durable for fires – *guardian of flame*. This strength is reflected in the image, which is not unlike the backbone or spine of man.

Eoh reflects strength, durability, and resilience. In simple terms, it is our *backbone* and what that represents metaphorically and symbolically. The connection with the earth and support of the roots would reinforce these features, but in northern culture it also reflects the connection to heritage and the ancestors, possibly because of its longevity. It is a useful rune to use in bindrunes for magical purposes.

* "Yew is the greenest of trees in winter; it is wont to crackle when it burns." (Norse)

** "Bent bow and brittle iron and giant of the arrow. (Icelandic)

PEORTH (P)

A Game

Peorth is a source of recreation and amusement to the great, where warriors sit blithely together in the banqueting-hall.

The meaning of this rune is problematic, and we do not have recourse to the Scandinavian poems for help here. If the pairing aspect of the runes is considered, then as the preceding rune **Eoh** represents the yew tree it could be postulated that this **Peorth** may represent a tree as well, maybe a deciduous one because of its shape. *P* is not a common letter in Old English, making it somewhat obscure.

However, this shape could represent other things, such as a gaming-cup (for dice etc.), or even a womb. The potential sexual implications are obvious. The womb implication has more significance when we look at **Beorc**, and **Peorth** can then be seen as an *open* representation of that rune. The impression of a womb or creative container is strong, and reminiscent of the athanor, or cauldron of alchemy; the container into which the base material for change is placed, to be worked on by the attendant alchemist as a reflection of his or her own personal and spiritual transformation.

The overall impression here is fruitfulness and change. This is reflected in the gaming association, which is indicative of chance and luck, hence the flux of life and also change again. Luck is an important concept that relates to a function within the soul in the northern mentality; in fact, it is directly named as a component in what I refer to as the 'body-soul complex' of the heathen worldview.

The word *blithely* indicates a casual or cheerful indifference, something northern warriors were renowned for in battle. If they died in battle they were transported to the great banqueting-hall of Valhalla, assisted by the Valkyries, and this may represent a level of kenning also present in the rune. *Blithely* can also mean improper, which might also refer to behaviour in the *banqueting-hall*; but I wonder – thinking about **Peorth** as feminine, womb, and the nature of the image itself – whether there is a libidinous and sexual level to this rune.

The overall impression is of change, flux, and the vagaries of the soul, and with it their acceptance in our lives. In this respect, the connection to the concept of fate or wyrd is profound. If paired with **Beorc** then **Peorth** reinforces the feminine quality of the soul as a journey through life involving birth and rebirth, nurturing and death. Whilst death is not overtly present here, it is inferred, and is found as an undercurrent in many of the runes.

Accepting what we are given in life and making the most of it in the colloquial but also the spiritual sense, **Peorth** may represent a challenge to the soul and our personal development. Having said this, the poem indicates a lightness and playfulness that contrasts with the serious business of warriorhood and complements it. In this respect, warriorhood can be a metaphor for work, occupation or other life obligations. **Peorth** might also infer that sexuality is a hidden part of the overall picture and one that needs including.

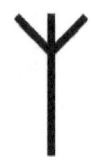

EOLH (X/Z)

Protection, Elk-sedge

*The Eolh-sedge is mostly to be found in a marsh;
it grows in the water and makes a ghastly wound,
covering with blood every warrior who touches it.*

Eolh is a challenging rune. At one level its meaning seems relatively obvious as protection to threatening forces; but if consideration is given to the representations of it that occur elsewhere in the Futharks, then a more complex picture emerges. There are some similarities here to how runes like **Thorn** or **Os** differ between the Old English and Scandinavian representations, and their respective meanings.

In the Younger Futhark, the rune glyph of **Eolh** is used for **Man**, where the meaning of the 20th **Man** rune of the Futhorc and Elder Futhark is also incorporated. There is no direct Scandinavian poem representation here, because these are applied to **Man**; however, I will refer to them because of this overlap. This is hardly surprising, as the shape strongly suggests a man with arms raised, or even the splaying of the first three fingers of the hand; one an act of supplication, the other more of protection.

The act of supplication in the religious sense is not emphasised in the rune poem, although the word *augmentation* is used in both versions of the Scandinavian poems related to **Man**. I think this aspect has been somewhat overlooked, and see this rune also to be one of prayer, dedication, and generally of a more sacred nature in word and action.

For example: It is energetically powerful to stand with feet shoulder width apart, arms raised up and outstretched at 45 degrees, as in the **Eolh** rune. This can be extended to a 'charm of protection' by saying, *Eolh Weardath Me* (OE and pronounced "EH olch – 'ch' as in 'loch' – WEH-ar-dath may"), meaning "Eolh protect me".

But the rune poem says otherwise. Here, as is a feature of the Futhorc, **Eolh** is reduced to a literal and somewhat floral perspective. Certainly, the elk-sedge is a sharp plant that grows in marshland and can inflict a wound if grasped. One extension of this is seeing the elk-sedge as a boundary plant, not unlike a hedge, and often symbolising the marginal or liminal existence of the magician who lives in the world beyond and which the hedge affords protection for. This being the case, the *blood* of *every warrior* may have a deeper shamanic and initiatory significance.

However, the elk as animal is ignored in the Futhorc, and probably overlaps the magician kenning as a shamanistic power animal, as the Elder Futhark refers to it directly. Closely connected to the horse in northern culture and having regal and spiritual significance (particularly if the horned stage – the horned god – is considered), the elk is an animal that in the wild seems to walk the boundary between the physical and spiritual worlds. It therefore affords a protection of a different but overlapping kind.

As indicated, this reduction of elk to elk-sedge is a pattern of movement of the image and meaning from the Elder Futhark to the Futhorc, whereas I believe it is relevant in the understanding of the full importance of **Eolh**. Added to this is not only meaning of protection, but also the spiritual aspect of surrender, or letting go. There are similarities here between the image as a man and the figure of the crucifixion, after all. I am a little surprised this is not emphasised in the poem or elsewhere.

SIGEL or SIGIL (S)

Sun

The sun is ever a joy in the hopes of seafarers
when the journey away over the fishes' bath,
until the courser of the deep bears them to land.

All three of the rune poems refer directly or indirectly to the sun — but not the moon — in an obvious manner. The image could be seen as a ray of the sun and, when doubled, is known as a svastica of Indo-European descent, meaning *to be good*. As we know, this meaning became inverted by the National Socialist Party, or Nazi movement, of the 20th century.

The power of the sun is identified in the Norse (*I bow to the divine decree*) and Icelandic poems (*destroyer of ice*); the latter may refer back to the **Is** rune.* ** The sun had significance in the north and often had a feminine attribute; possibly specific to the goddess Freo/Freya, who wept *tears of gold* in a grief state. In another version, her tears became amber when they fell into the sea. Amber was also seen as *the tears of the sun*, referring indirectly or symbolically to her tears. The cyclic variation of the sun becomes more pronounced the further north one progresses, making the female gender association increasingly understandable.

In the poem above, the indication is that the sun was an important feature to the seafaring peoples of the north (*the fishes' bath* is a metaphor for the sea), particularly when it is considered how far they ventured and expanded prior to Christianisation.

The *courser of the deep* may refer to a horse and journey, as exemplified in both earlier and later runes in the Futhorc, but also metaphorically points to spiritual assistance on life's journey.

The sun indicates not only the spiritual world, but also to its manifestation within this world without recourse to any intermediary god or goddesses; that is, apart from the consideration of Freo (and she only indirectly). In modern language, **Sigel** is a direct connection with the higher self. The name itself may also refer to a *sigil*, being an inscribed symbol having magical power, which is how this rune symbol is often used in the form of an amulet.

Sigil is a powerful, direct, and magical rune. Although in the modern era we see it as masculine, this has not always been the case. The femininity of our core spirituality; our direct and cyclic relationship to it; and the association with gold (also the culmination of the alchemical process), and even grief (in wounding, trauma, and healing) reinforce its power and intensity.

* "Sun is the light of the world; I bow to the divine decree." (Norse)

** "Shield of the clouds and shining ray and destroyer of ice." (Icelandic)

The **Hagal** aett: As a whole, this aett seems to fall into two equal parts. The first four runes appear to be a continuation of the creative process of the first, **Feoh's** aett, although much more on the human plane. Then there seems a change in tone, marked by **Ger**. Although a modern interpretation, I have found it of interest to assign each of the first twelve runes to a month, starting with **Feoh** coming after winter.

My sense is that this aett is one of individual creation, manifestation, and an evolution that extends to the following – Tir's – aett. The first three runes, being an extension of the first aett, seem to define an individual's existence. Then there is a progression of conception to birth and coming into existence as the *higher self*, which will make the next aett interesting reading.

Now to Tir's aett:

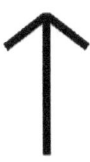

TIR (T)

The God

Tiw (or Tir) is a guiding star; well does it keep faith with princes; it is ever on its course over the mists of night and never fails.

In the rune poem designated as **Tiw**, which is an alternative spelling, the rune **Tir** represents the god who lost a hand to the wolf Fenrir, a monstrous animal that threatened all of mankind as well as the gods. The loss was a consequence of the trade-off that kept Fenrir chained, and therefore not a threat to the peace and tranquility of the Aesir (gods), as well as indicating Tir's role in justice. You may want the check out the myth to see how he ultimately lost his hand!

Tir is referred to as the *one-handed god* in both Scandinavian poems, indicating again the more profound mythological connections existing in those cultures.* ** With Thor/Thunor and Woden/Odin, he is one of the big three of the northern pantheon. The reference to *smiths* in the Norse poem is a little enigmatic and I wonder if this refers to an artificial hand being made, as this is a significant theme in heathen mythology. Similarly with *princes*, and specifically *prince of temples* in the Icelandic poem. This might relate to a religious function that **Tyr** fulfils; as a god undertaking a sacrifice for the greater good, this theme should not surprise us.

Tir is a sky god as indicated in the poem. Rather like Uranus and his usurper, Zeus, in Greek mythology, he was ultimately superseded by Woden during the Viking migration age (800 – 1100 CE). Both are gods of war, although Woden adopted this with his other functions, leaving Tir as the god of justice. The runic image does seem to lend itself to phallic interpretation, although this does not appear a distinct feature of the god; like Zeus, this sexual aspect was more the province of Woden.

As a sky god, **Tir** would seem primordial, though in our time he presents a more humanised face, which is a characteristic of the ensuing aett that is often named after him. As the rune poem indicates, he is the god of justice, predictability, and order. From an inner perspective, this implies honesty and integrity, the moral imperative in man. Hardly primordial; so, are these later editions, or an indication of something prior, beyond history in the culture that sustains?

Tiw is the alternative rendering of **Tir**, resonating phonetically in our day of Tuesday. Similarly, Wednesday is Woden's day, Thursday Thor's day, and Friday could be Frey's day... or maybe Freo, Freyja or even Frigg's day, if we are being democratic from a gender perspective!

Intuitively, I wonder if **Tir** may relate to the fir tree? It is easy to see the graphic as phallic or a weapon, but it also looks like a fir. Trees are relatively common in the Futharks, gods are indirect (as are the sexual references) and later we come across weapons, although not in the Elder Futhark. Is the fir, the tree that first populated the landscape of the north after the glacial age, resonant with **Tir** as an older god? I suspect that this is the case.

Tir represents justice, and the image even looks a little bit like the so-called scales of justice, as well as being 'upright'. Certainly, there are moral values implied here and these are present in the poem. But there is also something further, even lost (like **Tir's** hand) in a deeper balance or connection with the potentially world-destroying wolf, Fenrir. It is as if beneath the justice there is something immense that is threatening, even unto destruction.

I am a little surprised there is no Christianisation in the poem, as the graphic and its meaning remind me of the deeper significance of the crucifixion. Maybe the message of **Tir** is to be careful about using misplaced or false values to protect ourselves from forces that might otherwise be overwhelming, and to genuinely ask ourselves what is right or just sometimes in the face of collective values and ethics that may differ. There is a thread of implied courage here, as well.

* "Tyr is a one-handed god; often has the smith to blow." (Norse)

** "God with one hand and leavings of the wolf and prince of temples." (Icelandic)

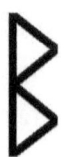

BEORC (B)

Birch

*The poplar bears no fruit; yet without seed it brings forth suckers,
for it is generated from its leaves.
Splendid are its branches and gloriously adorned
its lofty crown that reaches to the skies.*

The reference here is to the poplar tree and this is supported botanically in the poem; however, the imagery could also point to the birch, after which the rune is named. It is fertile, vigorous and plentiful, and the reference to 'skies' may associate it with the preceding rune, **Tir**. It could even be seen as **Tir's** complement when gender is explored.

The gender as well as fertility is implied in the image itself, which is distinctly feminine, whichever way you look at it. This shows a level of complementarity to **Tir**: god and goddess, sky and earth, male and female. The sexual imagery is deeply embedded here and not to be ignored, although here in **Beorc** this is woman and all her power. Reference has been made earlier to a possible association to **Peorth**, as with complementary breasts and womb, which further reinforces this interpretation.

However, the reference in the rune poem is to self-generation (*it is generated from its leaves*) and is implied in the imagery, as indicated. This points to our inner capacity for reproduction, as in the union of our complementary inner genders. There is a sense of spring and abundance, and of a tree reaching up to the sky. The almost cosmic imagery is further supported by reference to the *lofty crown*, which paints a regal picture in addition to the canopy of the tree.

The Scandinavian poems do not have the richness and abundance of the Old English poem, which may indicate a climatic difference and the relative richness of the British Isles, as indicated in the Icelandic poem.* In the Old Norse poem, the reference to *Loki was fortunate in his deceit* is very enigmatic, which I wonder about in reference to the different trees implied in this rune, and may also include the fir.**

Loki is the master trickster, maybe pointing to a level of kenning not yet appreciated in the rune. My suspicion is that the play between masculine and feminine, as in the two trees as well as other implications that I have outlined here, may point to hidden mysteries, maybe of a Tantric nature. This would be no surprise to me, as sexual and erotic images and interpretations permeate the runes, if the surface is scratched sufficiently, and would present no psychological conflict to the Heathen peoples from whom the runes evolved.

All this notwithstanding, **Beorc** is about deep and self-contained feminine energy that is capable of regal appearance and aspiration, even to reaching the sky. There are resonances here of the ascent of Shakti to and union with Siva in Hindu mythology. This energy is subtle and contained, sexual and erotic, yet strong. It is fertile and implies beauty, so irrespective of Loki hovering, it is quite optimistic and may be simply that every cloud has a silver lining.

* "Leafy twig and little tree and fresh young shrub."

** "Birch has the greenest leaves of any shrub; Loki was fortunate in his deceit."

EH (E)

Horse

The horse is a joy to princes in the presence of warriors.
A steed in the pride of its hoofs,
when rich men on horseback bandy words about it;
and it is ever a source of comfort to the restless.

The horse has been touched on in several places to date. In the **Eh** rune the relationship between the horse and its rider is fundamental, and even symbolised within the image itself. In fact, relationship itself is embodied in this rune, which could be seen as two horses nuzzling noses, or a couple walking hand-in-hand.

Without doubt this man-horse relationship was of historic and military significance, and hence its importance, being a feature of Indo-European peoples. It should be remembered that the fantasy image of the centaur is derived from this close relationship, possibly by observers who being unused to riders on horses, saw the two so interconnected as to be one being.

Yet there are levels beyond the literal, as the horse represents power and the relationship to it that is not seen with other animals in the runes. To harness the power of the horse requires a delicate balance between the rider and steed, which may add another level of kenning to *princes* and *rich men*. In this respect, the horse could represent not only the body, but also be a symbol of the soul.

The reference to *warriors* and *restless* gives the impression of forces beyond the immediate comfort of the poem. Whilst a warrior seemingly implies the immanence of battle, could it refer to the spiritual aspect of warriorhood? And could restlessness be the anxiety we experience when disconnected from our spiritual source? These possibilities maybe remind us not to read these images evoked in the poem simply at a literal level.

In shamanism, the soul of the shaman often explores the Otherworld in the shape of a *power animal*, often unique to the individual shaman. Of course, this need not be a horse, but it is a strong image of this relationship and the journey that is to be undertaken by the shaman. It should be recalled that Woden/Odin had an eight-legged horse, *Sleipnir*, upon which he traversed the various worlds in a vertical (spiritual) rather than in a linear manner.

Of further interest, mythologically, shamanically, and enigmatically, is that Sleipnir is the product of the union of the sexual union of Loki – in the form of a mare – with a stallion. The myth involves the building of the walls to protect Asgard, the home of the Aesir, and is worth checking out.

An intriguing aspect is that the glyph of **Eh** can also be seen as **Lagu** and its reflection, as in water. This can represent relationship with one's self, as in the myth of Narcissus, or the deeper relationship – via the medium of water and the art of skrying – with the great spiritual unknown. So, beyond the masculine imagery and its connection with Woden, maybe this is more his magician aspect and his relationship to the feminine, and hence Seith magic and its mysteries.

The horse **Eh** represents our power at different levels and involves a differing concept of control; more one based on cooperation with the unknown or spiritual dimensions. Too much control and we can kill the spirit of the animal, too little and it can run amok; it would seem to be all in the balance. There are similarities to **Rad** here.

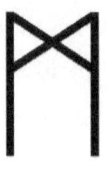

MAN (M)

Man

The joyous man is dear to his kinsman;
yet every man is doomed to fail his fellow,
since the Lord by his decree will commit the vile carrion to the earth.

Man could also be seen as a doubling of the **Wyn** rune and so contain some of its attributes. This continuation may be reflected in the first line, which reinforces man's divine connection, but does not continue through the poem, which in all sources indicates his mortality. Also, with the preceding **Eh** rune, the **Man** rune would seem to create another pairing or dyad that is a common theme in the Futharks.

The paradox continues in the Scandinavian poems that, whilst reinforcing man's mortality, also see him as *adorner of ships* in the Icelandic (recall the longboats of the Vikings) and the *claw of the hawk* in the Norse.* ** Although this latter reference could indicate his mortality (*augmentation of the dust*), it may have a shamanic reference. It is also the only place in the immediate rune literature where a bird is mentioned until we get to the extended version of the Futhorc, which I find of unexplained interest.

The Old English rune poem is – once again – laden with Christian reference, with *vile* indicating not only man's deprecated status, but also his potentially inherent evil nature (after all, evil is an anagram of vile). There is also the word *doom* used again; in this context it is an indication of his mortality, his impending death.

Is there something deeper here that the Christian darkness judges and obscures? In some respects, the rune can be seen as blatantly erotic and, if a doubling of **Wyn**, represents a sexual coupling. The rather obvious Christian influence here, as with all runes, can be removed to reveal a more magical level, particularly if the god/shaman Woden is involved (as **Wyn** would imply).

All in all, **Man** is a representation of exactly that: Man in his totality, inclusive of his sexuality; with his connection to the gods, but also his fragility and mortality. I use the word man here to include woman and, indeed, the image itself symbolically reflects this gender duality.

We are a unique composite standing between the worlds of the gods and creation, as is readily seen in the mythology of all peoples, and reflected in our psychophysical totality of body and mind or soul. We also have an awareness of our inherent gender duality, we all man and woman, both. The inherent 'dance' in the **Man** rune sees these apparent opposites as mirrors, reflective of each other and inherently connected as a unity, as in the Yin-Yang symbol; indeed, **Man** could be seen as the western equivalent.

* "Delight of man and augmentation of the earth and adorner of ships." (Icelandic)

** "Man is an augmentation of the dust; great is the claw of the hawk." (Norse)

LAGU (L)

Lake

The ocean seems interminable to men,
if they continue on the rolling bark
and the waves of the sea terrify them
and the courser of the deep heed not its bridle.

Here is one half – the left when looking – of the **Eh** rune, reinforced by the *courser of the deep*, with the word *bridle* confirming that this phrase represents a horse, a symbolic sea-horse. By contrast, and maybe without the same connection to the **Eh** rune, the Scandinavian poems seem gentle and even innocuous. Only the Norse poem provides some symbolic depth with a *waterfall* and *ornaments are of gold*, which may refer to 'tears of the gold' and hence amber; it would also connect this rune with Freo/Freyja and the feminine.*

The *bark* reference comes up in the **Iss** (Ice) rune of the Icelandic poem, with *bark of rivers* and even *roof of the wave*, indicating bark in this context to be the froth and foam of the wave. ** Whilst bark could refer to a tree (indeed, one dictionary definition relates it directly to **Beorc**) it could also indicate the noise, as in the bark of a dog that is made by the waves.

Overall, the English poem provides a challenging, even terrifying view of the ocean. In the poem, this is particularly so if the courser heed *not its bridle* and indicating, once again, the dynamic balance existent in nature and man's role within it. This does, of course, as already discussed, reinforce man's role in this balance, although in this image he would seem to be at the mercy of the elements.

Although not directly in the poems, the word *lagu* is related to the Germanic word for leek. With garlic and onion, this plant was considered to have magical properties; indeed, they are all considered to have strong and pervasive healing qualities. Additionally, the leek, as with the image itself, has a strong phallic quality. This is seemingly at odds with the image as sea, lake, and hence the feminine. However, there may be other associations here that enforce a more complex erotic symbolism.

Specifically, and from a magical perspective, the sea, lake and water represent the maternal matrix, or the womb. The lady of the lake is an image from Celtic spirituality that reinforces this image, and provides a complex, even sexual symbolism for the casting of Excalibur. This aspect of the rune may foreshadow the Grail elements that emerge in the rune extension to the Futhorc. Water is also used by magicians, most specifically witches, for divinatory scrying, reinforcing the feminine nature of **Lagu**.

Lagu is the deep feminine in her mythological, magical and archetypal context, beyond the simplicity of the mother's womb. The images are wide and complex, sexual and mystical, but overall (and with the association of Freo) point to the Vanir and the magic of Seith. **Lagu** may also indicate a letting go of the self (or ego) into the waters of the collective (maybe with a little magical encouragement); to see what emerges from the depths, that may be significant and guide us forward in life's quest.

* "A waterfall is a River which falls from a mountain-side; but ornaments are of gold." (Norse)

** "Eddying stream and broad geyser and land of the fish." (Icelandic)

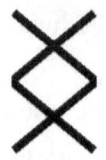

ING (NG)

The God (or Frey)

Ing was first seen by men among the East-Danes;
till, followed by his chariot, he departed eastwards over the waves.
So the Heardingas named the hero.

The rune **Ing** is also an ancient god of the land, rather than the earth per se (a feminine function), and may be paired with **Lagu** as land-water. This would also pair the god Ing with Freo, which occurs in other myths in his guise as Frey. Ing is fundamentally a fertility god, as is Frey in his pairing with Freo, with all the attendant sexual implications. The similarity of the glyph with the modern representation of DNA is notable; did these cultures have a depth of appreciation about life that we have only recently rediscovered?

The image can be seen in several ways. As an enclosure, it indicates containment as of a race or people. As a seed it is fertility, both of semen and the egg, and with the association to Ing and Frey, and hence Freo. In the rune rows it is also a seed, as its shape manifests in a lot of the runes.

Ing can be seen as an overlapping and reflective doubling of the **Kenaz** rune of the Elder Futhorc around the vertical axis. It is also a doubling of **Gyfu** around the horizontal axis, so reinforcing the meanings associated with that rune. Turned 90 degrees to the right it could be a pictograph of a couple making love, viewed from below.

The Ingvaeones, one of the core Germanic tribes involved in the Anglo-Saxon migrations, also lived close to the sea. The *East-Danes* could be the Swedes. The chariot is an image that often refers to the skies and maybe a constellation of stars. The *Heardingas* are a royal line of East Anglia. Whilst these associations expand on the rune poem with a historical flavour, I am not sure whether they add much in terms of magical meaning.

There are no other poems to explore the meaning of **Ing**, as it is not present in the Younger Futhark. Because its relationship to, and potential pairing with **Lagu**, would make this feasible. Does the rune that follows it in the Younger Futhark – **Yr** – replace it? By the meanings of **Yr** in the Scandinavian poetry it would seem not, as this relates more to the rune of the same name in the rune extension. Does **Ing** represent a deeper stratum that has been negated and excluded in the Viking era? Has Galdor magic superseded Seith?

As an aside, **Ing** clearly demonstrates the problem of the glosses, distortions and other obscurities that the rune poems create. I have nominated these as being mainly Christian, so why include them? Because they are part of the Futharks' history and their development, and it is not necessary to exclude them to unearth the deeper more mystic-magical layers. Also, this inclusion is important when we move beyond the runes of the Elder Futhorc into the extensions that developed and existed within a Christian framework of progressively increased influence.

For the magical import, we can return to the prior comments, where the **Ing** rune is the fertility of the land and represents a seed, even semen. Separately, and in combination with **Lagu**, there is a lot of encoded imagery that relates to Seith magic, but also the fertility of the land in the agricultural cycle and their mutual interconnectedness from the Heathen perspective. The erotic tone of this rune is strong. These are all deeper understandings of the relationship of the genders, but also of 'man' with the land and sea; in this it is a rune for our times and our genuine relationship to not only others, but also the environment.

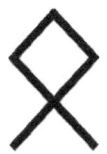

ETHEL (OE)

Inherited Property

An estate is very dear to every man,
if he can enjoy there in his house
whatever is right and proper in constant prosperity.

Ethel and the rune that follows, **Daeg**, are somewhat interchangeable in their relative positions at the end of the Germanic and Scandinavian Futharks. There are arguments for and against what the order should be, as would be expected with such a variation and ongoing question about it. This variation exists nowhere else in the Futhark, although it is present in rune extension in the Futhorc, to which we will come. I will simply adopt the order as given in the Old English rune poem, and not enter into the argument; as neither rune is represented in the Scandinavian rune poems, these cannot be drawn upon for assistance.

There is general agreement as to the meaning of this rune in the common and literal sense. Having pictographic and ideological similarities to **Ing**, it represents not only individual land or estate, but also tribal lands, extending to the idea of heritage across generations. In this sense, the rune image can be seen to be a boundary, a fencing of owned land.

Ethel is common in naming, particularly of a compound nature (for example, Ethelred) where it appears to have an association with nobility, as the word *Atheling* means *prince*. Over time it has been more commonly used as a girl's name, which is an interesting psychic shift of note. An additional image is of a ring, symbol of inheritance, kinship or even kingship. An archetypal symbol of the self, the ring is a powerful image of ownership, containment, and power. In this respect, the image of **Ethel** is like a [wo]man (many of them are, you may have noticed) in a balanced posture.

All the above can be, of course, a metaphor or metaphors for the individual in an inner manner. In other words, it relates to genetic heritage, ancestry, and its manifestation in the world. The idea of a boundary is also relevant, in a relative manner, to how a man conducts himself in the world. The term *right and proper* and the word *prosperity* link the **Ethel** rune to many others in the Futhorc, with the by-now familiar Christian overtones that permeate this poem. Interestingly, it associates moral values with wealth, or implies a less material to *prosperity*.

Ethel has pictographic similarities to other runes, such as **Ing** and **Gyfu**, as well as **Ken** in the Futhorc. Often it is worth reading a rune in combination with those it is graphically and hence symbolically related to, as I indicated earlier with **Ethel** and **Ing**, but also extends it to others in anticipation of the comments to follow.

Whilst at a more obvious level **Ethel** relates to ownership and inheritance in ways described, it is the boundary I find significant, as this implies protection against threat. On an inner level, this is protection of self or even genetic heritage against wounding and trauma; a shamanic function as with a shaman. Maybe this is why the King was always strongly associated with the Druid for counsel in the past (mythologically, think of Arthur and Merlin).

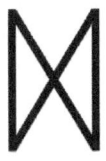

DAEG (D)

Day

*Day, the glorious light of the Creator, is sent by the Lord;
it is beloved of men, a source of hope and happiness to rich and poor,
and of service to all.*

The **Daeg** rune of Day is commonly represented as two right-angled triangles facing each other nose-to-nose. This image, however, is of the 24-hour day as day-night and the cyclic flow between the two. Indeed, this may be a hidden or lost feature of other runes, such as **Sigel** (sun-moon) and **Ger** (summer-winter), in that each name latently and paradoxically contains its opposite.

An alternative version of the pictograph extends the two vertical staves in both directions. This then makes **Daeg** look like two facing **Thorns**, or even **Man** with a little downwards slippage of the middle 'X', recalling **Gyfu**. It may be interesting to explore the connections between these three runes further, particularly if one or other occurred with **Daeg** in a reading.

There is little literal here in the poem (we lack input from Scandinavian poems here); the Christian influence I hope you can now recognise as being particularly strong. As elsewhere, I often wonder what is hidden or excluded in this process. In the absence of natural or agricultural reference, the rune would seem to refer more to the day as *light* in the spiritual sense. That the image inherently contains the opposite (*darkness*) is of particular interest in this Christianisation process, which has excluded it.

However, all this does not stop the spiritual connotation of light being of divine origin and the great leveller; that is, it can bring *hope and happiness to rich and poor*. Also, inherent in the poem is the **Sigel** or Sun rune, which closes the aett and indeed the whole Elder Futhark on a light and spiritual note.

Daeg does not appear to have the excitement or magical import of much of the Futhorc. However, it may be appropriate, as indicated, to see it in relationship to both **Ger** and **Sigil**. This would give it ritual importance, as well as being important to the agricultural cycle and hence our relationship to nature and the environment. From an inner perspective, **Daeg** indicates day and night together; that a man is whole only with his shadow integrated. In any reading, maybe the shadow, as well as the light, would be given a clear focus.

The **Tir** aett: **Tir** has a much lighter quality than the second; particularly the first half beginning with **Hagal**. In some ways, this supports the theme of the Futhorc to date (and in the Elder Futhark) being divided into two sequences of twelve, as the last four runes of the **Hagal** aett connect with the **Tir** aett in a similar manner to the first four connecting to the **Feoh** aett. Anyway, this is speculative; there was a great emphasis on the number eight in the north, being the manner in which the year and its attendant ceremonies were divided, but I suspect there is a significance in the twelve as well, possibly astrologically.

Certainly, the **Tir** aett is more related to man and his relationship to the land and earth. However, the magical and spiritual elements are metaphorically (at least) present in all the runes, as well as permeating the Futhorc to date as a whole. It will now be of interest to see how these insights flow into the extended Futhorc, with restricted guidance from the Old English rune poem, and now with more emphasis on our own individual insights and associations.

The Rune Extension of the Futhorc

The extension of the Futhorc may have been a natural development to cope with phonetic developments in language by the Anglo-Saxons in their new homeland, prior to the wholesale adoption of the Roman alphabet there, as well as the co-existence of these two languages over time and the influence of the indigenous – Celtic – culture.

As stated earlier, I have generally avoided significant reference to the phonetic development of the runes. At the most immediate level this is because I believe there is too much emphasis on trying to relate – or even equate – the Futhorc to the Roman script. That this can be done, to a relative sense of completion, there can be no doubt. But this does not equate the two and gives the erroneous impression that the Futhorc in some way is simply a language that can be equally well, or even better expressed through Roman script, and therefore more easily understood.

Some of this phonetic understanding is relatively impossible anyway, as we are not absolutely certain how the spoken word was employed. It also lends itself to a relatively modern habit of taking a word in modern English and doing a kind of reverse transliteration. If this approach is going to be adopted at all, it is wisest to first translate the word or words from Modern to Old English, and then transliterating. If this was done at the time, it would be a better and more accurate approximation.

My concern here is that this literal approach diminishes the other dimensions to the Futhorc; being the metaphoric, symbolic, imaginative, magical, and spiritual dimensions. These are progressively reduced in the Roman script and almost completely absent in Modern English. Seeing the runes in their own light assists this process, because even the scholarly material does not point to such a conflation; in fact, it usually does the opposite.

All these comments notwithstanding, the initial extension to the Futhorc appears to be primarily phonetic and therefore trying to accommodate language changes and development. It is here, maybe, that the Futhorc parts company with the more esoteric trends in the Elder Futhark, as represented and reinforced by the Younger Futhark somewhat later. In this earlier stage (around 500 CE) it may be that the Futhorc was seen as a written language before being superseded by the Roman script. The later development of the Younger Futhark in the Viking era, several hundred years later, may then be seen as some sort of return to a magical authenticity.

Following the change in the phonetic meaning of the **Os** rune (where the 4th rune of the Elder Futhark becomes the 26th of the Futhorc, which with the variation in the 6th **Cen** rune together accounts for the name change from Futhark to Futhorc), these changes were to accommodate the varied vowel usage and being **a, ae, y** and **ea**. These are present in the inscription of the Futhorc on the so-called Thames sax (a 9th-century knife found in the Thames River in 1857), although the rune poem brings in **Io/Ia** – a slightly enigmatic rune as we shall see – between **Yr** and **Ea** at position 27.

The names and meanings of runes 25 to 29 are closely related to the Celtic and the indigenous Ogham script, probably used for communication and magically. However, rune 29, **Ea**, although a vowel, like its four predecessors, feels more related symbolically to the last four runes 30 to 33. The Old English poem stops at rune 29.

The last four runes (30 to 33) are consonants that rarely occur in inscriptions, but are present in manuscripts. These are collectively called the Northumbrian rune row that originated around 800 CE, and which has a mythic or symbolic significance that indicates a reconnection to an evolving spiritual context in the runes. This is in quite a different manner to the Elder

Futhark's contraction into the Younger Futhark, as well as the actual spiritual content and orientation. It is notable to me that this follows the Synod of Whitby, where the Roman Church assumed religious control of the Christian Church in Britain.

As before, I will leave further research of the phonetic aspects of the runes to individual pursuit, as they take this exploration in a direction largely incommensurate with the magical and spiritual usage I am espousing.

This ongoing sequence is sometimes referred to as the fourth aett:

AC (A)

Oak

The oak fattens the flesh of pigs for the children of men.
Often it traverses the gannet's bath,
and the ocean proves whether the oak keeps faith
in honourable fashion.

The clear meaning here of **Ac** is of the oak tree, strong and hardy. The two principal uses of oak were of its fruit, the acorn, as pig food, and as the most resilient wood for the building of ships, so vital to the seafaring Germanic peoples.

This would have related to those peoples of the south and west, including the British Isles, as the oak does not grow in places like Iceland and the extreme north of Scandinavia. This fact alone differentiates the Futhorc within the Futharks and identifies it more with the Anglo-Saxons, and maybe their relationship both with the Celts and England.

The rune poem contains only the second bird reference, although it is metaphoric: here it is *gannet's bath* for the sea, seemingly in preference to the *fishes' bath* as mentioned earlier in the **Sigel** rune. The difference is that birds like gannets catch fish, so changing the emphasis.

The image is a slightly truncated **Os** rune, which connects it to the gods, although more specifically to Thor/Thunor with the strength and power of the oak. The oak has a magical quality that is revered amongst the Celtic peoples and their priesthood, the Druids, the religion that the Anglo-Saxons usurped and probably incorporated; however, Christianity does much to obscure this process from the underlying Heathen perspective.

Although it would take us too far afield, it is with **Ac** and the runes that immediately follow it that there is a perceived continuity between the runes and the Celtic Ogham indigenous to Britain, prior to the arrival of the Anglo-Saxons. Ogham is sometimes called the 'Celtic Tree Alphabet' and may have originated in Ireland. It is based on 20 glyphs that represent trees and here with **Ac** that the overlap with the runes is more pronounced, and with the initial runes of the Futhorc's extension.

Ogham has also been associated with the Celts' priesthood, specifically the Druids, as the script is considered a cipher. I suspect that these early runes of the extension indicate a connecting point and overlap between the two scripts, irrespective of the differing views of their respective origins that flow into the obscurity of prehistory.

In these respects, and from a more magical perspective, the **Ac** rune represents power, and specifically power of the magical will. Symbolically, the image is of a man holding a stick or wand, as would a magician, with a bit of phallic overtone. This is reinforced by other features common to the oak, such as being steadfast, resilient, and courageous; all features of the good magician.

Ac calls for strength and endurance, and complements the **Ur** rune in many ways. As such, it is a rune of healing; dealing with the projections of others in a creative and magical manner. From this perspective, **Ac** relates more to Woden and a different spiritual perspective to Thunor.

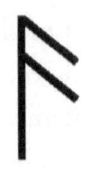

AESC (AE)

Ash

The ash is exceedingly high and precious to men.
With its sturdy trunk it offers a stubborn resistance,
though attacked by many a man.

This 26th rune of the Futhorc has taken on the image of the 4th rune of the Elder Futhark, **Ass**. Indirectly, **Aesc** has also taken on some of **Ass's** characteristics with the latter's change from the Elder Futhark to **Os** in the Futhorc. The ash tree is characteristically that of Odin/Woden, as it was on the ash, which may have been the world tree Yggdrasill, where he hung for nine days and nights in his shamanic discovery of the runes, or specifically the rune charms, within the well of Mimir where he attained their inherent esoteric wisdom.

The similarity to oak is indicated in the shape of the rune, as well as the closeness phonetically, specifically around vowels and their subtle variations. With this phonetic similarity between **Ac** and **Aesc** the connection with **Os**, and therefore indirectly to the Elder Futhark's **Ass**, it is worth considering these runes and their meanings as a kind of interconnected complex, maybe with further levels of kenning not directly revealed.

In the poem, these common features continue, although *attack* is a little unclear, it may simply relate to the ash's exploitation and usage by man. Alternatively, if the ash represents Yggdrasill, the world-tree of Norse mythology, then it is under attack from its roots being perpetually eaten by the mythical worms that gnaw at them.

The meaning of this rune overlaps that of **Ac** considerably, although the associations to Germanic mythology remain quite strong. The ash is also synonymous with the making of spears rather than bows, a fact that has considerable association with ritual sacrifice. The glyph itself can be seen as a spear or a barb. Spears and sacrifice emerge as distinct themes later in the rune extension, and it is towards these features that **Aesc** is possibly directed. This may be a feature of this triad of runes more generally, as the overlap on indigenous and prehistoric spirituality (the Celts and Druids), though directed toward some more historical spiritual themes that become evident in the rune extensions.

With the conflation of these similar shaped runes across the Futharks, and within the Futhorc itself, it is difficult to see **Aesc** in isolation. There is also some association symbolically with the **Eoh** rune, although there it is a yew tree that appears in the next rune. In fact, it is worth seeing these three runes in some sort of continuum, and maybe indicating a convergence of ideas with the indigenous spirituality that the Anglo-Saxons met in England.

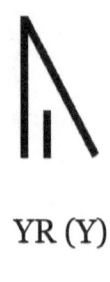

YR (Y)

Yew bow

*Yr is a source of joy and honour to every prince and knight;
it looks well on a horse and is reliable equipment for a journey.*

Yr is yet another tree rune, reinforcing their importance in the Futhorc as compared to the Futhark, as well as the connection to indigenous British spirituality. The yew is represented in the 13th rune of the Futhorc, **Eoh**, but the difference here is the reference to its use as a bow, which it pictographically resembles. The yew rune of the same name in the Younger Futhark, **Yr** the 16th and last, makes combined reference to the tree, bow, and arrow: *"Bent bow and brittle iron and giant of the arrow."* (Icelandic poem)

The first line of the poem indicates its significance with *joy and honour*, and hence **Wyn**; the second line associates with two other images and known runes, being the horse and the journey, **Eh** and **Rad**. There is therefore quite a range of interconnections between other runes of the Futhorc by virtue of the poem, whereas the glyph would associate it more directly with **Ur**.

The bow and arrow is reliable equipment to take on a journey and for use in hunting; its use possibly precedes even the origin of the runes. It is also able to have an impact over a long distance, which may be its symbolic and magical relevance, in addition to its use as a weapon. Of further interest is that the image is that of the **Ur** rune with an arrow inside, so the attributes of **Ur** would also be relevant here. There is even some phonetic overlap here between these two runes.

It is difficult to give a separate meaning to **Yr** and the comments at the end of **Aesc** are also relevant here. The symbolic and magical meanings seem at one level obvious (strength etc.), but may represent a subtlety or magical meaning now lost to us or present in Ogham. This is reinforced by the connection between the respective runes of the Futhorc and Younger Futhark by name, even if the image differs.

However, the Younger Futhark image of **Yr**, which is an inverted **Eolh** from earlier in the Futhorc (or **Madhr** in the Younger Futhark), reminds me of a crossbow. But maybe of greater significance is that **Yr** is an inversion of the earlier rune **Madhr** in the Younger Futhark. Reflecting this inversion in the Futhorc, **Eolh** is inverted in **Calc**, which we will come to later in the rune extension. To my mind, this negates the use of runes in an upright or inverted position for readings, which I see as a modern addition to the tradition.

My deeper feeling is that **Yr** is metaphorically pointing toward the significance of the runes that are to come (and maybe specifically **Calc**), as there is a hint of an alchemical nature with the *brittle iron* reference found in the Icelandic rune poem for **Yr**, which we have already looked at with the yew rune of the Futhorc, **Eoh**.

I tend to see a distinction between the above three runes and the two that follow. The reason for this I trust will become apparent as we progress:

IOR or IAR (EO or IO)

Fish, Eel or Serpent

Iar is a river fish and yet it always feeds on land;
it has a fair abode encompassed by water, where it lives in happiness.

This is a strange beast, literally as well as symbolically. Literally the meaning of **Ior/Iar** is uncertain: a *river fish* that *feeds on land*? It is apparent that an eel may well fit the bill, but it is by no means clear that this is the case. Maybe here there is a 'watering down' – please excuse the pun – of the dragon or serpent from the intensity of the Germanic myths to a more acceptable image in Old English; after all, this is a frequent feature in the Futharks.

From the symbolic perspective, backed by the rune poem as well as some etymological gymnastics, I would favour **Ior** meaning a serpent, even a sea-serpent. Serpents, worms, and dragons abound in Germanic mythology; and the rune image, although with a striking resemblance to the Younger Futhark **Hagall** (hail) rune, looks serpentine enough to me. The primal power and intensity of this rune seems present in the image, but lost in the poem.

If this is the case, then this rune is slightly out of context with the three before, and the one that follows, that make up the 29 runes of the poem. Maybe, in this case (and as some commentators think) it should follow the next rune, **Ear**, and bridge to the more mythic Northumbrian extension to 33 runes. My own impression is that it marks the end of this sequence of three runes, rather like **Ger** does in the second aett. That would make **Ear** (the next rune) more part of the Northumbrian extension of runes 30 to 33, in spite of the fact that it has a verse in the Old English poem, where the others do not.

In the magical context, the serpent is a strong sexual image that recalls the kundalini energy coiled at the base of the spine, evoked and awakened by ritual sexual activity. It is one of, if not the, primal energetic power in the human psychophysical organism.

There is a sense with **Ior** of balance and equality, with the gender-ambiguous nature of the serpent. Yet the serpent, or snake as kundalini, is the primal force of our spiritual evolution where the male and female elements are also in balance. This may be the prime feature of **Ior**, balance in the primal sense, as reinforced by its home in the waters of the maternal womb.

EAR (EA)

Earth, soil

*The grave is horrible to every knight,
when the corpse quickly begins to cool
and is laid in the bosom of the dark earth.
Prosperity declines, happiness passes away
and covenants are broken.*

With the possible exception of **Ior**, and if the Thames sax is considered, **Ear** is the final rune of the Futhorc as defined by the sequence of the rune poems. It therefore represents finality, with some degree of dark imagery and pessimism: It is not a cheerful rune. With it, the body passes away and disorder once again supervenes as *covenants are broken* with a slow decline according to the forces of disintegration and entropy.

However, the decay is not just physical in the poem, it is also mental, emotional, and social; it cuts across a wide spectrum of meaning. Although seemingly related to personal death, the images also recall the mythic Ragnarok of Scandinavian myth, the so-called *twilight of the gods*, where everything passes away, somewhat cataclysmically, and foreshadows a new beginning. In this there are some remarkable similarities with Christian belief, as well as Woden's self-sacrifice on the great ash tree Yggdrasil, recalling the earlier Futhorc rune of **Aesc**.

This is not a rapid death, it is one of decomposition, and reminds those familiar with alchemy of the sombre stages of fermentation and putrefaction. These stages mark the transition from the consolidation of the individual, or conjunction of the soul in the *lesser work*, with its transition to the spiritual *greater work* if successfully negotiated.

In this respect, **Ear** has distinct parallels to the crucifixion and resurrection; indeed, the image of this rune could well be a man suspended on a cross. If so, and my intuition is correct, this marks a sequence into these latter runes of the Futhorc, which contain a merging with the mystical aspects of the Christian influence, and with the remarkable unifying themes of alchemy to guide the process.

Although **Ear** is about death, the poem paints a gloomy picture. But in the Heathen Mentality, this is not the case; death can be seen as a transition, either as a metempsychosis or to a more glorious existence, as exemplified in the image of Valhalla. **Ear** is the death that marks the ritual dismemberment and burning at the beginning of the alchemical process that is reflected in shamanism, as well.

Ear marks the end of the Old English rune poem and most extant versions of the Futhorc. However, there are four further runes, derived from what is known as the Northumbrian rune row and preserved now only in manuscript form, that are particularly worth considering. Without them **Ear** would be leaving the Christian story at the crucifixion and not considering the resurrection. Modernity sometimes makes a similar mistake, and here the more mystical inclination of Northumbria is significant, at least in my way of thinking.

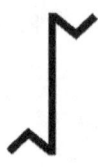

CWEORTH (Q)

Ritual fire

Cweorth is the ritual fire of change and transformation. It complements **Nyd** in many ways, although here more as the receptacle of the fire initiated in **Nyd**. The image could well be of flames leaping up into the air. As cremation, it is the liberation of the spirit from the body. In ritual initiation, and as commenced in **Nyd**, it is the completion, the transformation. In many ways, this is an extension of **Nyd** in terms of process, yet also and more particularly that of **Ear**. There may also be some resonance here to the torch of **Cen**.

Of further interest here is that the rune glyph of **Cweorth** is also that of **Peorth**, with the lower part of the stave a mirror-image of that part of the rune. The name is similar and even complementary; phonetically it is P and Q. This may provide insight into the **Peorth** rune that was previously lacking; is it a fire container, an oven, or an alchemical athanor (vessel or crucible)? And is that why **Peorth's** meaning is difficult to appreciate in the context of the Elder Futhark? The images of this rune and **Cweorth** both have an 'as above, so below' quality about them; this phrase is a core one drawn from alchemy.

In alchemy, the 'prima materia' – the base material to be transformed – is placed in a container called an athanor, as we have discussed elsewhere. Then heat is applied and the process of transformation initiated. Is this the next stage from the somewhat alchemically-flavoured death of **Ear**? Is this alchemical process mirrored in the runes **Peorth** and **Cweorth**? Plenty of questions, but I find them rhetorical, because I do see the answer in the affirmative. I think there is more to be considered here, which these questions bring to light for exploration; a process that itself is part of the alchemical process.

Cweorth indicates a process of change or transition that succeeds **Ear**. It is clearly delineated in the alchemical process and indicates a difficult, life-threatening but also a life-changing transition, which demands support rather than protection from these forces. It is a powerful image that, to my mind, reinforces much of the pathways of spiritual evolution that are symbolised in the crucifixion and resurrection, and hence reinforcing the progressive Christian influence in these latter runes from a more mystical and esoteric rather than an exoteric perspective.

But this is Christian influence now devoid of the poem, and in contrast to the verse in **Ear**. This sheds some light on the tone and quality of the poem, which I have drawn on at many points earlier in the Futhorc. We are at some relative disadvantage without a corresponding poem; but maybe also the imperative is to return to the image, name and symbol, and draw the sort of conclusions being elucidated here without the religious influence. Maybe we are getting back to the alchemical and mystical source that underlies the religious message … maybe beyond death to not only resurrection, but also a pathway to spiritual realisation?

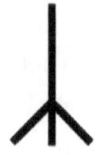

CALC (K)

Cup, Chalice

Obviously, **Calc** is an inverted **Eolh** rune, the 15th of the Futhorc and Elder Futhark. In the Younger Futhark there is a direct correlation with the 16th and last rune, **Yr**, the yew bow. As this 16th rune marks the end of the Younger Futhark, it can and does relate to death (as does the yew tree itself). There are resonances of the death association here with the inversion of the cup image, and the chalice association is a portent of the death of Jesus, as well as the mystery of the Eucharist. In this respect, the more mystical stream of Christianity via the Holy Grail is hinted at.

Obviously, as can be seen above, the rune name **Yr** of the Younger Futhark is matched in rune 27 of the Futhorc, which then takes a different shape, akin to **Ur**. Although seemingly a little confusing, this cross-fertilisation between the various rune patterns indicates a dynamic interchange at various levels of kenning, also seen elsewhere in the Futharks.

What interests me most about this rune is that it seems associated with the two before and two after by way of sequence, but bears little resemblance to the runes of the Elder Futhark or the first 24 runes of the Futhorc. That this rune has strong associations elsewhere and most particularly with the Younger Futhark is intriguing. Given the latter's reputation as a more magical rune row, I wonder about the cross fertilisation here with Northumbria across the North Sea.

In all these connections and associations death is not a final act, but a transformation. In the Germanic tradition, the drinking horn would serve a social and religious function as well, and parallels much of the Christian imagery. Here are points of merging and connection that indicate a creative flowing together of these changing times, rather than seeing them as fundamentally adversarial.

Although I have hinted at the connection between the previous rune, **Cweorth**, and **Peorth** in the second aett as an alchemical container, it may be that this is the function of **Calc**. Being adjacent to **Cweorth** and with the dyadic theme that periodically permeates the Futhorc, this is an additional possibility. However, there is also the sense that this is of a higher order of transition or spiritual evolution. There is also something in the name. Calcination is a stage – the first – in alchemy. It is the stage when the base material is placed in a container, which is then closed, and then fire applied to it to effect change.

One interesting observation here is the simple fact that **Calc** is actually an inverted **Eolh**. This inversion peculiarity is seen here in the Futhorc and the Younger Futhark indicating, as discussed earlier, that the modern habit of seeing a meaning in readings where runes are inverted would not have been a traditional one. This particular inversion may therefore have been of more magical and mystical import, and relate **Calc** back to **Eolh**.

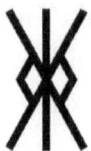

This is an alternative form of **Calc**, sometimes referred to as a **Double Calc**, or **KK**. I have put it here next to **Calc** although it is by no means certain that is its place; maybe it should be separate, or even put to the end of the sequence because of the similarity to **Gar**. I will leave the question of place open, but point out that it does satisfy many of the qualities described in **Calc**.

This **Calc** is a deep image and indicates that the alchemical transformative process is proceeding in a spiritual manner. As a chalice, or even the Grail, transubstantiation is both a physical and a spiritual process; born of sacrifice, it is entering into the 'kingdom of heaven'; or, in Heathen terminology, Valhalla.

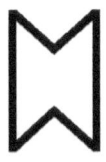

STAN (ST)

Stone

Stan is a familiar term in the Anglo-Saxon world and persists in the modern era in male and surnames. The wider association to stone is indicative of stability and a grounded quality, which the image itself presents. Indeed, it could be a rune stone, or symbolise the use of stones for inscriptions. It may also harken back to the Stone Age and the heritage from there that flows through the Futhorc.

The image could also be seen as an enclosed **Peorth**, adding another level of mystery to that rune and its possible further connection with these latter runes of the Futhorc. Certainly, there is a sense of potential energy within the image with all these associations.

Continuing the alchemical theme is the concept of the 'stone of the philosopher', which is the base material – the prima materia – and is the beginning of the alchemical work to ultimately become the 'philosopher's stone'. This somewhat confusing and paradoxical terminology is common in alchemy and reinforces its reputation as being somewhat obfuscatory. This resultant philosopher's stone is believed to catalyse the transformation of base metals into gold, as well as being the 'elixir of life'.

This latter association provides a connection of **Stan** with **Calc** and the Holy Grail, as well as the ultimate outcome and completion of the alchemical process. What is intriguing is that the stone is central to the art of alchemy and its association with the transformation images and myths of Christianity and the Grail Legends. Why is this? Alchemy would seem to be a very metallic art with the various materials used, and its associations are with the planets and astrology. Yet the whole process is centred around the philosopher's stone.

Historically, the various Iron Ages that encompass the period of the runes followed the much longer Stone Ages. In prehistory, the erection of great circles and other monuments with huge stones was a distinct feature of the time, and with ritual, ceremonial and other religious functions, including the life and death cycle. What is the nature and continuity of the stones? Are the remnants of this significant in gravestones and our attraction to gemstones? What wisdom have we lost?

Although rhetorical, such questions intrigue me. It requires an intuitive and psychic disposition to approach them and the territory embraced in the runes. It is what draws me in, because not only do these latter runes, including **Stan**, intrigue me about the past, I suspect they have more to yet tell us about our time and the future.

The final 33rd rune could be considered part of the fourth aett, or on its own:

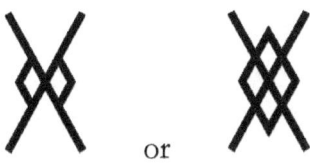

GAR (G)

Spear

Mythologically the spear rune is that of Woden and is representative of Yggdrasill, the world-tree. It is also the spear which marks part of Woden's self-sacrifice to obtain Galdor, the wisdom of the word contained in the runes. This, as well as the image itself, tends to mark **Gar** apart from the other runes that precede it, although it also remains symbolically connected.

Gar is somewhat enigmatic as well as being complex. It has no direct associations, particularly phonetically; the letter G is, after all, the **Gyfu** rune. From the Christian perspective, the spear used as part of Jesus' sacrifice also comes to mind and illustrates that this may be a rune of self-sacrifice. Psychologically it may represent the death of the ego, but in spiritual or alchemical terminology it may be the ultimate transformation of matter into spirit.

The image itself may be seen as a complex bindrune, in either of the given representations. These alternatives are provided here for the sake of completeness, as sometimes one and then sometimes the other is used by different commentators. In either form is a contained image that is quite like a mandala in appearance, and could also represent the unified self in the psychological sense.

It contains within itself much of the imagery of the runes that precede it, and orders them into a unified whole; although the **KK** version of **Calc** would better serve this function, and is sometimes put in this last rune position of the Futhorc as an alternative version of **Gar**. It is certainly a better alternative to the so-called blank rune suggested by some modern rune-makers to serve this psychic function.

Different commentators provide alternatives around the **KK** version of **Calc** and the two of **Gar**, given here, even to the point of having further numbers to the rune row, such as the 34 and sometimes built around these three and other variations. In the past, I had seen the **KK** version of **Calc** as the final rune, because of its inherent complexity. Now I tend to see it with either version of **Gar** as complementary, as spear and chalice, placed around the alchemical stone. The spear and chalice, it might be recalled, are central icons in the Holy Grail legends. Their presence here in the Northumbrian part of the rune extension may be no accident.

What might be appreciated from this – although disliked by some – is the obvious Christian influence that has permeated the runes through Northumbria. Historically this is perhaps no surprise, and the Christian influence should definitely be seen as mystical and esoteric, hence the profound association with alchemical imagery. This is reinforced by the Holy Grail references I have drawn upon here. But, more than this, I believe that the continuity of these spiritual pathways within the Futhorc is a testament to the connection between the Heathen and esoteric Christian traditions; sometimes and too often seen as being in conflict.

Gar as a symbol of a spear is quite a challenge, and one that reinforces the sacrificial motif. The element air predominates in this rune, and – although a little far-fetched – could the image also represent the bellows that fans (inspires) the alchemical process? A symbol of the descent of spirit into matter maybe?

Addenda

There follow some brief comments on the subjects of Christianisation, sexuality and magic, which have arisen as a result of this examination of the Futhorc. The Christian position has already been examined, but will need further focus as we move more into the spiritual context of the runes that includes Christianity, but extends beyond (in terms of Heathenry) and beneath it (in terms of esoteric or mystical depth), so here in this section are some bridging comments. Similarly with sexuality and magic; these areas will have increasing prominence as we move forward. There will inevitably be some overlap, but see this as reinforcement rather than duplication, as these areas are sometimes difficult to digest and integrate.

On Christianisation

I have made frequent reference to this, most notably in my comments about **Ing**. As stated there, I have opted to not only include the Old English poem as a reference and guide, but to explore it to some extent in the text about each rune. I could have opted otherwise, particularly as the poem is a later addition to the Futhorc in the latter part of the first millennium, when England was deemed Christian.

However, this process was gradual over time – several centuries – and would also have been a kind of *top-down* process. By this I mean that it was expedient for religio-political and not necessarily spiritual reasons that the ruling classes adopted Christianity, so this would have filtered down through the population only slowly over time. Indeed, the Heathen undercurrents remained present for much longer. They are considered to be a factor in the Witch Hunts of the Mediaeval period, and they permeated medicine not only then, but continue to do so.

My emphasis here has been to try and unravel the deeper meanings of the runes, rather than see the Christianisation process as oppositional to the deeper more Heathen and magical meanings. Why? Because there was really no battle, as evidenced by the Celtic Church and the Northumbrian influences. Christianisation was a dynamic and integrative process, as well as having oppositional components.

Also, when it comes to the esoteric and mystical threads, I argue that there is no significant opposition. So, the process is to unravel the religious (exoteric, political etc.) rather than the mystical threads; because these latter were – and are – present in Heathenry. This is one reason for the acceptance of Christianity, as the *Good News* was literally that.

All these points become increasingly relevant and evident as we move into the rune extensions to the Futhorc beyond the Elder Futhark, and will be further explored.

Sexuality

The gender emphasis on the male, in spite of any rhetoric about the term really referring to man-woman, is actually quite remarkable. Not only is it blatant and indicating little in the way of gender equality, it also points to the Church as a political and socially-controlling tool, acting in support of whatever vested interests were to its advantage. For a Heathen society noted then – and still now – for its more gender egalitarian position, this is significant.

There is also enough in the content of the runes for me to see that there were times when a woman should be nominated, irrespective of the man-woman argument. Were women seen as such a threat in runes like **Cen** and **Lagu**? I believe they were. And that this suited not only political stances, but also associated functions like healing (and hence medicine) and magic. More to come.

It would be interesting to take the runes and see them from an exclusively sexual imagination, and of course, I have done this. There could be many other facets to this, such as: education; ritual; fertility rites; association with nature and the agricultural cycle, and of course magic. In these respects, the runes are practical and instructive, maybe governing intimate life of the family and community. There would also be controversial features, like open sexuality and orgiastic functions, particularly in ritual and ceremony, as well as shamanistic ones – healing, divinatory, and prophetic.

Magic

In the northern traditions, there are two branches to magic, Galdor and Seith. With what has been covered to date, the reader should have a reasonable appreciation of them as the two gender-based disciplines with their respective roles in the culture of the time. There are images of both in the public imagination, but it is Seith that is the more distinctive and controversial. Given that Woden learnt Seith magic as part of his initiation process is very significant, although the runes themselves fall more into Galdor magic and Woden/Odin's initiatory sacrifice on the World Tree, Yggdrasill.

Although Christianity can be seen to be controlling in its religious context by suppressing the body and sexuality, more broadly it does this by suppressing woman. But not only this, it is, by its very origins and nature, decidedly patriarchal. What this means is that other functions of the masculine would come under its suppressive scrutiny. Woden being initiated into Seith magic and the gender-bending implications of this is a case in point.

Magic is also intimately involved with healing. Add to that the separation of the soul, the distancing of heaven and the fear of death to a people not used to such worldviews, then healing taken up by a patriarchal medicine (and predominantly Mediterranean as well), adds another level of obfuscation and control. Magic is left in the margins it would seem, although it was more integrated before the turn of the millennium, and particularly the events of 1066.

Yet it did not die out; it is – like sexuality – with us still.

Sample Readings

What is being undertaken with a reading? It is a psychospiritual inquiry; entering into a dialogue with something ultimately indefinable, though commonly referred to as *God*. But there is a subtle difference here, as it is not the same as *praying* where the intercession is with some sort of great, more powerful force or *entity*. Praying is a passive process, but also the entity is distinct and considered to have an independent existence. This is not dissimilar to the receptive manner in which many approach the dreaming process. Some would consider this position as fundamentally *mystical*.

More controversially maybe, a different position is where the individual – you – are a part or facet of this greater entity or reality, although simultaneously and paradoxically superseded by it. This reality – both physical and metaphysical – is something we can more actively engage with: A petition becomes a dialogue. Ultimately, this is the basis of the many ways this reality, or the divine, can be related to or dialogued with … be it divination or a magical process of some kind. I prefer to call this entity, reality or divinity the *Ground of Being*. Somewhat ironically, I am using a term by the Christian theologian, Paul Tillich. In contrast to the above, this process is more *magical*, because it considers the individual intimately involved in the process and, to some degree, having an authority and determination in the dialogue and hence the outcome.

So, where do the runes fit in? It is worth remembering that in Norse mythology, the runes are a gift of the gods. Odin received them in his self-sacrifice on the world tree Yggdrasil, as a tool, means, or language with which to communicate or dialogue with the gods. So, it is as if this language – both literal and symbolic – is something *god-given* and we learn to use them in a ritualised reconnection process to appreciate in a greater, expanded and more holistic manner the nature of our query ... although, ultimately, the interpretation is our own. And within this, lies a great responsibility.

To the practical demonstration: I have made my own Futhorc. I have a selection of flat slate pieces that I use for making runes. I continually add to this collection, from various sources, and I experiment with styles of engraving and inscription, as well as making differing sets. For example, I have an Elder Futhark made from river stones sourced in central Australia and a Younger Futhark with runes carved on slate.

The Futhorc I am using here is also made from this slate. The particular set I have used for these readings was made in a ritualised and creative process. I have used an engraving tool to carve each rune shape into the slate, and have then used my own blood to stain and empower it in an initiatory manner. The runes are kept in a pouch specific for ritual purpose and rune readings for myself and others.

A Rune for the Day

This method is described in the Divination section and is the first method outlined there (p30, above).

This morning (in 2013) I took the rune pouch and put my hand inside. I then 'felt' around the runes, sight unseen, and drew one that seemed to attract me.

It was **Ior**:

Some prior reflection:

I had slept deeply following a meeting I had had yesterday with my colleagues, where, amongst other things, we had discussed this book. As this meeting was on a Sunday it had also created a little domestic disruption, but I was also determined that what I see as my emerging more mythic direction – and my commitment to it – be primary in my life henceforth.

When I drew **Ior** the first thing that struck me was that I had chosen a rune from the runic extension of the Futhorc; I had determined beforehand that on this day I would write the *Rune for the Day* in this book with whatever rune I chose. This followed a recent discussion with one colleague about how to complete the book with the sample readings.

Ior speaks to me of core or primal energy, undifferentiated and sexually androgynous. I associate the rune with fire and the primal energy of the dragon. At present my own sexual energy feels quite remote, yet I felt quite strong and powerful at the time I drew the rune, so maybe this is indicating creative energy? I take the reading this way, and prepare for my day accordingly.

My understanding of the rune was that it indicated to me a confirmation of the direction I had opted for. My core energy is craving this transition, and I have been particularly entranced by the runic extension to the Futhorc and its spiritual significance in the Northumbrian runes. As this rune is, in some ways, a transition to this extension, it is both a confirmation and also a clear indication that some of my core interests – sexuality and gender issues – need to be the foundation and taken into this further inquiry.

A Divinatory Reading

This method is described in the Divination section and is the second method outlined there.

Being in the groove from the above *Rune for the Day*, I now decide – as I am actually writing this – to do a reading to provide some clarity and an orientation of my work with the Futhorc project from here, and specifically into Anglo-Celtic magic, medicine, and spirituality.

I am apprehensive and find myself prevaricating... but it is time to stop typing and draw the runes:

ᚱ ᛟ ᛋ

I am immediately drawn to the middle rune, **Calc**, then I look to the runes on each side, which are more familiar to me from my earlier Elder Futhark days, to gain a little context. Without reference to any text, I am gaining an initial impression, so I will now go and have a cup of coffee and contemplate them a little before writing further ...

The first rune, **Rad**, is a familiar one. In the present context, it may indicate a progression from the *Rune for the Day* I conducted earlier today, but also indicates to me the beginning of the next stage with all the inferences contained in that reading. I am also drawn to the delicate balance here between my intent and the forces I am dealing with, some of which – sexuality and gender – are embedded in **Ior** as well.

Rad is leading me toward **Calc**, a rune with which I am less familiar, so I look at my own reading with more intuitive attention than usual. Again, I have drawn a rune from the runic extension, although this time from the Northumbrian extension and without a rune poem to guide me. I think this reinforces my commitment to using the Futhorc runes, but also that this rune particularly highlights the death and transition – even transformation – of the process I am presently involved in; essentially it deepens it.

In terms of content, the image of the Holy Grail has interested me for many years: over a generation ago, I had considered interrupting my medical career to write a doctorate thesis on the Grail. The fact I didn't do so may indicate I wasn't yet ready or mature enough; maybe I am now, and maybe it also indicates my interest to be in this transitional time, when mystical Christianity was extant and now sadly lacking in our era. Is this a task for me? A process I am destined to be involved in? I look to the last rune as it might help me.

Eoh indicates *strength, durability, and resilience* and *reflects the connection to heritage and the ancestors*, according to my own reading. The connection to the body and the spine particularly reminds me of the comments around kundalini energy I made to the **Ior** rune. The image of the bow may point to a more distant future that I may be involved in, as represented by the yew and extending from my own ancestral heritage. The death image is also present, continuing from **Calc**; this seems to be a time of great transition for me if the outcome is not to be literal – maybe I have no choice but to follow the wyrd that the runes have lain out for me.

The three runes can thus be connected. The first is where I come from, what is now behind and beneath me. I have begun and am on a journey, driven by powerful forces and with spiritual intent. The second rune tells me where I am now presently positioned. It points to my spiritual interests being the core of the challenge that faces me and with which I now have to work. The third rune is the direction I am going, the future. I will require strength and resilience, but also this is a marathon and not a sprint; maybe a legacy even beyond my own life here.

Collectively these runes point to challenges of my ancestry and heritage, rather than to personal issues. In the light of what preceded the question, I would also take this reading back into that context, as it will help me define my role and direction within this collective enterprise. At a deeper level, I believe it is directing me toward a clear avenue of my spiritual pursuits and their creative expression; although the depth of the transition and the spectre of death is something to take account of in this process.

To reinforce this reading, the three runes could be combined into a bindrune. To do this I take the vertical stave of each rune and superimpose them. The individual attributes are then placed around, as if the runes are stacked one on top of the other: there is a cross on the lower left-hand side, with **Rad** showing clearly to the right. The resulting pictograph may capture other runes; in this case, there is **Gyfu** with the cross (and maybe a Christian reinforcement), which appears to be supporting **Rad** as the main thrust of the bindrune, thus indicating the importance of the journey rather than the destination.

Postscript

I have taken these readings from my earlier work, written several years ago. Some months after this time, and when the earlier work *Just Add Blood* was being completed and submitted for publication, I went through a strange windy and stormy winter's day in my study. I will never forget the day, I felt immersed in the weather in a way I had not before; it was both disturbing and also invigorating. It was like Woden was present and my world outside was in upheaval, although I was content in the comfort of my study.

That evening, I went to collect a takeaway Chinese meal and, clearly for the first time in my life, felt beyond any fear of death. It was a surprise and also a relief. Then my work as a medical practitioner began to become strange, or I was estranged from it. Things started to unravel, and I felt powerless to stop this process. There was something strangely familiar about what was happening, although it culminated in a rapid decision to leave practice, voluntarily and absolutely.

Just Add Blood was published, but I did not feel it to be the backbone I was looking for. Instead, I negotiated my path away from practice and its familiarity, attempting to find some stability. This process took a few years, until I started to return to this work, which I did when I started to explore the concept of the *Soul* from the Anglo-Saxon perspective. I started to feel strong again, and began to work on this book and complete what I had started all those years ago.

In addition to modifying and including *Just Add Blood* in this current book, I am completing my long-awaited work on the Grail, entitled *The Charm of Making*. The runes of this time were maybe more prophetic than I had accounted for then!

From this point on, all that is written (with the exception of some of the *Postscript*, as well as the *Appendices*) is new material, drawn from these intervening years and the paths I have gone down. What was then a simple reading appears to have followed me down the years and foreshadowed a deeper pattern governing my life. I feel now, more than ever, that I am in the realm of **Eoh** and that things are now moving forward according to my wyrd and reflected in the reading.

On impulse, I draw a rune in the present:

ᚹ

So, maybe I am on track!

Medicine Wheel Reading

This method is described in the Divination section and is the third method outlined there. I will also use this reading to explain this method further, which I did not do at the time of writing *Just Add Blood*, as I was somewhat hesitant about using it in this strictly written and therefore limited context. Time moves on, so I have decided not only to do a reading according to that method, but also to use it to explain more about the *sacred circle* and *medicine wheel* from my own perspective.

There has been a recent change of emphasis in a relationship I am involved in that may be setting the tone for this reading. The question is whether my anticipated direction from this point portends stepping more definitively into the psychospiritual and creative context I have been developing for myself, in spite of external demands, or even because of them.

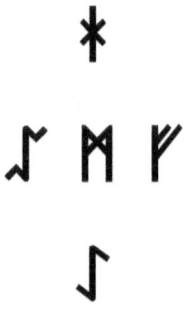

Man is the central rune that I drew. This is central both to my initial question and also to the outcome. It is tempting to associate this to the interpersonal relationship I described, not forgetting that it also relates to *inner* relationship, which I see the outer one representing, as a projection in the world. So, any question I have about this interpersonal relationship are a reflection of the one I have with myself.

The remaining runes are drawn starting in the East and being placed sunwise or deosil (being anti-clockwise here in Australia) at the compass points in a cross around **Man**; being successively; **Feoh, Ior, Cweorth** and **Eoh**. Of significance to me is that the runes **Ior** and **Eoh** have appeared in the earlier 2013 readings, immediately above. I refer to the comments made there, particularly around the connection between the two that I came upon in the second reading. These runes represent the North and South respectively, which I see as the more spiritual poles of the circle, masculine and feminine respectively.

In effect, I see the North-Centre-South to represent my psychospiritual totality, as represented by the spine and the Kundalini energy of **Ior** that arises from **Eoh** and passes through **Man**, which now, more definitively, represents the masculine-feminine dyad within myself. Whatever I am seeing in the interpersonal is a reflection of the intrapsychic, a projection, if you will. There is a progression from the grounded strength of my ancestry and tradition that is engaging me and challenging my purpose and direction; it is also feeling quite a solitary (ad)venture.

Feoh in the East is a challenge. The East is traditionally the place of the masculine, youth and power; the latter two being distinct characteristics of **Feoh** with the exception that this rune is distinctly feminine. I see this as the source of my power in the current question; it is in the feminine operating through the masculine portal; my Soul in action. Conversely, in the West is **Cweorth** the alchemical *ritual fire* of deep change and transformation, and in the feminine position of passion. Together with **Feoh**, this is a very soulful combination, yet one that is undergoing a change... but to what?

I return to the centre and **Man**. The transformation is one of taking the male-female polarity in the world, evaluating and valuing it more deeply and internal, leading to the alchemical reunification of the masculine and feminine through the fire of transformation. It appears I have a major challenge in front of me, and it is within me. The events of the outer are simply a reflection of this process, and I should not confuse them. It would be maybe an easier path to see them in the world and not within myself, as this may avoid or even negate the intensity and potential sacrifice that this transformation demands.

I have done this reading sight unseen, and elucidated it as I wrote above; a kind of divination-in-action or psychic channelling. I will leave it unedited and as a testament to this process being alive and real in the metaphoric or even symbolic sense. It has moved me, and given me a clear feeling of my direction from here.

There are many more associations I could have added to each of the compass directions, both in isolation and in their connection to each other as a medicine wheel. I have drawn on this knowledge in an inspired manner to write the above; it would take me too far afield to go into detail about this. After all, I have written about this in an instructive way elsewhere, in *Sacred Space*.

Postscript to the 33 Rune Futhorc

The Futhorc

This section is a brief discussion of some of the points raised as we travelled through the Futhorc, mainly for some increased elaboration and clarity, even if there is a little duplication. Most of the points raised here will become the subject matter of a more detailed analysis that will follow this section regarding the significant influence in areas such as sexuality, magic, medicine, and spirituality.

By now, it is clearly apparent that my approach to the exploration of the Futhorc rune row is predominantly intuitive. There is no ready reading of "this rune means this", but a more interlaced and interlocking picture; a bit like a tapestry, I like to think. This can be seen with the frequent cross referencing to other runes, which those readers interested can readily easily extend upon, using the rune shapes and imagery as a guide.

The extension to the Futhorc contains some intriguing patterns. The initial runes 25 to 27 seem a furthering of the more familiar and natural images contained in many prior runes, with the emphasis on trees that may also relate to the parallel Celtic tradition of Ogham. Sometimes referred to as the Celtic Tree Alphabet, Ogham was also present in the first millennium of the CE, particularly toward the western regions of the British Isles.

In simplistic terms Ogham and the connection of the Celtic priesthood, the Druids, with trees is considered popular in our era and remains strong. It makes sense that there would have been a cross-fertilisation process with the Ogham and the emerging Futhorc, even an assimilation of the former into the latter over time and distinctive to the Futhorc, with its development from and beyond the Germanic Elder Futhark.

It should not be forgotten that these magical systems – and the Futhorc particularly with the present study – did not arrive out of the blue, but would have emerged from earlier proto-alphabets, language, and other more symbolic means of communication. This is suggested in various places here and I would hold it to be self-evident. It is also suggested by the linear progression of the rune row itself, where the more primitive and natural then becomes increasingly more symbolic and esoteric. This could also be metaphorically seen as a temporal flow from the Neolithic through to the Middle Ages.

Neither should the Christian tradition be ignored, and it is frequently referred to above. It is tempting to try and exorcise the Christian influence in the Futhorc to return to some sort of prior Heathen authenticity. But I hold this to be a modern fantasy, along with other New Age aspirations; it would be better to consider the process in its reality and entirety. Because I do not consider the Christian influences to have simply usurped or suppressed the prior Heathen traditions, but to have frequently and creatively merged with them, particularly if the more mystical undercurrents are explored.

The cunning ('kenning') amongst the Heathen magicians may well have adopted early Christianity as a method in the maintenance and further development of their traditional values; indeed, as a progression of them. They were not then as incompatible as we might perceive them to be in modernity. In that era and united by mystical threads, like the similarities between Woden and Jesus, there are many areas of commonality.

This overarching trend becomes more evident after the 27th rune. Rune 28, **Ior**, has some features that I have likened to the eastern concept of kundalini. **Ear**, rune 29, is more elemental with earth and transformative with its focus on death. The image also has features that repeat in **Cweorth**, rune 30, and **Stan**, rune 32. The elemental theme is also present in these latter runes; fire, water, earth and air are all there, if you scratch the surface, as is some of the more esoteric and symbolic imagery that extends from the elements; such as stone, spear, and chalice. The remarkable similarity here to esoteric Christian Tradition needs reinforcing, particularly with the proto-Grail imagery. This maybe foreshadows the development of the rich corpus that would emerge over the next centuries, following the closure of the Viking age and then with the creative emergence of the Arthurian myths in the next millennium.

I have also emphasised the alchemical themes and associations, which can be seen to connect to this trend and its development, yet also look back deep into pre-history, as do many if not all of the themes explored here.

That these later developments in the Futhorc occurred in northern England, which is why this sequence is referred to as Northumbrian, may not be a surprise. This region was the meeting ground of differing peoples and their influences. The Celtic Christian Church there was also suitably distant from Rome and somewhat distinct and idiosyncratic with, as I read it, a greater emphasis on self-determination in spiritual matters. It may not then be a surprise that it became a breeding ground for spiritual ideas that emerged in the succeeding centuries and influence us still, having deep roots in our indigenous pre-Christian spirituality.

Tradition

I have chosen a Traditional approach to the runes, but why?

There are modern versions available, such as Guido von List's attempt at the turn of the last century to unify the runes with

Havamal, coming up with an 18-rune sequence. There is also Ralph Blum's attempt to accommodate a rune for the so-called *Self* within the Elder Futhark; the argument for which I negated, particularly when **Gar** rune of the Futhorc was considered.

Yet I have deliberately chosen to link the runes back to Tradition. My experience is that we neglect Tradition at our peril and that any attempt at modernisation should stem – with some sort of continuity – from Tradition and its timeless and archetypal presence. It is debatable where Tradition exists with the runes, but we do have some basis to consider the above discussions to rest within it reasonably authentically. And, of course, it is further open to discussion as to how accurate this particular representation is; it is putting my personal imprimatur on the field, after all.

Certainly, there are modern variations in interpretation, particularly with phonetics. I am sure many of the apparent gaps will be filled in over time, and some of the more contentious areas clarified; however, it does seem that we have a fairly exhausted corpus to draw on in the absence of any further significant discoveries. Some aspects, such as how exactly the Anglo-Saxons spoke, will remain forever unknown, and some further aspects will be ultimately unknowable.

I am not espousing Tradition in some sort of regressive manner; it also exists in the eternal present. I just believe that it is important that any modern understanding of the runes – and other similar material from Tradition – should have some sort of continuity to remain authentic. Otherwise, it is very easy to introduce subjective and personal interpretations that have only limited validity; we see all too much of this in New Age spirituality, which has also tainted runelore.

Yet this is all in the service of advancing Tradition into the present and future. I contend that it is the loss of Tradition that leaves us somewhat rudderless in the modern era, leaving us lacking depth, and thus living in a kind of two-dimensional scientific and technological flatland. I am certainly not taking a regressive position here; I believe we connect back to Tradition, but with our feet in the present, and our vision toward the future.

This is more specifically the case where Christianity is losing its relevance in our time. When I initially began to explore the runes, I thought I would discover my Heathen roots and establish a reconnection. I certainly have done that; but I have also found that there is a Christian theme in the Futhorc that has embraced the more mystical spirituality of Christianity, and furthered it. It is this more esoteric undercurrent that I believe has significant relevance in our time as we reach the end of the scientific era.

Other Disciplines

Here I am going to draw on what is of primarily of interest to me and where it relates to my personal and professional future, as well as being significant to the material at hand. However, as I share this, you may find some resonance with what I am exploring.

The magical traditions have had a significant revival in modern times. But, as I have discussed in the text, I believe it is important to link this development with our heritage. I have found that runelore adequately fulfils this need. The above can be extended to magical practice in the operative sense, as well as ritual and ceremony; all sadly lacking in our times, when the magical *will* is somehow disparaged as mere psychological ego.

As a medical doctor, I am also fascinated that the Anglo-Saxon mindset did not have a mind-body dualistic mentality to health, but instead a more integrated vision that included the realms of superstition, magic, and the work of the spiritual. Academic inquiry has revealed that Anglo-Saxon is not merely a poor cousin to Mediterranean-based medical systems and is more applicable to our mentality, if this is your heritage too.

I believe these undercurrents have a lot to tell us about modern medicine and where it has gone astray by excluding this wider and spiritual dimension of mind. I will certainly be exploring these themes in more detail in the future.

The Religious and Spiritual Context

I have already referred to this area in some detail at various junctures. However, and at the risk of further duplication, I would like to put this significant background in a more definitive context. Why? Because it is an important one that cannot be ignored, and even though I have tended to minimise some other disciplines and their input, the religious and spiritual context is so fundamental to the runes that it cannot be ignored.

Speech, vision, and the dextrous use of the hand are three attributes that distinguish we humans from other species, relatively or absolutely. There are various imperatives for this development that go along with the development of the brain and nervous system, although the significance or evolutionary consequences of these may yet unfold and be beyond what we can presently anticipate. They link the senses and brain to our creativity and the spiritual realm. The runes take advantage of all three attributes in various combinations; so, like the creative and spiritual impulse with which they are intimately connected, they are a thread or stream in our evolutionary development – and a unifying one, as well.

In some ways, we may have overstepped or outstripped ourselves in this impulse, which makes us vulnerable as a species. It is my view that the emotional, creative, and holistic functions within us have been relatively sacrificed in this process; therefore, there is a need for their reinstatement of importance and reconnection, in terms of our physiological and psychological functioning and wellbeing. There are signs that this reconnection process is occurring, although the forces against seem apparent and sometimes overwhelming, in terms of such issues as wealth imbalance, climate change, political control, as well as the various theatres of violence and trauma, both in warfare and domestically. Vexing issues like drug addiction are better seen in this context rather than a rational medical and legal one.

This is by way of background to indicate that the exploration of our heritage and its traditions is not just some sort of psychoanalytic regressive fantasy, but an attempt to reconnect with lost psychic threads that we recognise still carry emotional importance and significance, particularly in healing. The degradation of language and written communication over the last generation or so, aided and abetted by social media, should highlight this concern. In fact, communication more generally is apparently deteriorating, adding to the family, social, and broader community breakdowns with their lack of ritual and ceremonial bonding, not assisted by a Church with lessening relevance and being scandal-racked to boot.

Which makes my focus on religion and spirituality a little paradoxical, until we uncover that how it exists now is not how it always was, and this includes neglected aspects of Christianity. I am not in favour of a Heathen worldview that denigrates Christianity in a wholesale way and believes all of its influence should be exorcised to return to some purist Heathen position. There is much in the Heathen way of life that reflects and mimics the aspects of Christianity we would condemn, but the reverse is also true, in that there is much in Christianity that reflects and mimics what is healthy and wholesome in the Heathen way of life. But how – and is it of any value – to distinguish them?

Let me put Christianity on one side for a while, before returning to this question, and go back a little further in time to ask about the origin of the runes. To this point, we can determine that the definitive rune rows emerged in the early centuries of the Common Era, but from what? Personally, I find this sort of approach reductive. It relies on various rational disciplines, such as history, anthropology and archaeology to make these determinations and then uses others to fill in the gaps.

By reductive, I mean that the conclusions are based on and limited by the hard, physical evidence we have to hand, whereas – rather like the discovery of the black swan in Australia, when only white swans were considered to exist – something could arise or be found that completely changes our view and restructures how the evidence fits. I believe something similar has happened in my field of medicine, such as with infectious disease in the recent past, and may happen yet with cancer. In mental health, it is also apparent that other disciplines may impact on the way we view it, such as sociology and religion. So, why not with the runes too?

What I will be inclined to do is something I apply to medicine generally and mental health in particular, and that is to take a broader more holistic view that also includes the unproven and speculative, to see if that gives a more complete understanding into which the hard evidence better fits, rather than getting tangled with experts, evidence, and academia, with all their vested interests. So, what follows is unashamedly speculative and, no doubt, much may be proven wrong. But equally, it may provide perspectives that encompass some of the more problematic areas more holistically and creatively.

It is unlikely that the rune rows that have presented themselves early in the CE are some sort of degeneration, mainly because from this point forward and evidenced by findings, there is an ongoing evolution process. It is also appropriate to compare this process with other written and language systems, as diverse as the Roman alphabet and the Ogham script. What we are lacking in this is much of the context in which the runes were used, such as language and communication, ritual, and specialised arts like divination and magic.

There also some broader issues to consider. Any runic *finds*, before the modern era, would have been associated with a hunter gatherer society, with agriculture coming in the latter period prior to the common era, at varying times and in different regions. So, how much does agricultural society reflect their development, and how much influence can we attach to the societies that preceded it? Because here we are in mythic territory, where there is no 'soft' evidence (runes etched into wooden staves, for example) and where what evidence there is, is combined with ritual process, as in cave paintings and on stones more generally.

A step back and we have the megalithic culture that built Stonehenge, where the mysteries still abound. Then we have the apparent succession of migrations and later invasions in Britain that characterised the post-Ice Age period some 10,000 years BCE. And was the Ice Age simply a climatic variation, or did it follow some sort of catastrophe such as a large meteor crashing into the planet? Were there civilisations before, intimated in the myths of Atlantis, that found some sort of continuity through this period? And before this, how much influence did the Neanderthals have, and maybe still have genetically on our spiritual development?

These questions remain speculative, but they do favour a view of the runes as reflecting a hunter gatherer society and its shamanic worldview that developed over many thousands of years, which was intimately connected with the environment and had a spiritual outlook that was seamless in and within daily life. There is also a feeling that subsequent agricultural society changed the role of the feminine in this respect, demonstrated by its inclusion in the spirituality and magic of the northern European peoples. There is much in the runes that reflects these societies and their intimate and varied connection with the environment.

This is not a book about shamanism or the spiritual belief

systems of these peoples, except to give a background and context to the runes and what they represent. They obviously have various levels of kenning, or meaning, many of which I have discussed. But there is something important here that needs to be expressed. Each rune is not simply an analogue of its meanings; in other words, it is not appreciated or understood on some sort of horizontal plane but also has a vertical one. For example, why is **Eolh** the shape it is? Is it because that shape when enacted physically, evokes some feeling of surrender, devotion, and hence act as a supplication for protection? I believe it does, and that this is true of all the runes. So, the reverse is true; *protection* can only be represented by this rune.

Now there are some problems here, such as with **Cen**, where there are different representations across each of the known Futharks; how is this to be understood? I would suggest that, with **Cen**, there are various facets too of a core ritual process involving – maybe – wounding, death, enlightenment, and sexuality. Is **Cen** then a rune in its own right, or a *seed* rune for others, or both? Do later runes like **Calc** attempt to integrate these facets, as well as adding in **Eolh** in some sort of bindrune? Does this indicate the spiritual profundity of **Calc** as the chalice of the Holy Grail?

In a roundabout way, I have come back to Christianity, so let me address my feelings about it and its influence in the present context. It must be obvious to you by now that I do not see Christianity and the Heathen path in any sort of binary black-and-white way. If the Druids were the ruling priestly class at the time of the Roman invasion, then their decimation is more attributable to this in a lot of England (although not Britain, more generally); however, I suspect the Druids survived, adapted, and modified themselves over time. And when Christianity came to Britain in the wake of Rome's conversion, then they adapted and integrated here, too. But why?

Because esoteric Christianity tells of the Good News. And the figure of Christ is prefigured in their religion; most certainly is this the case with the Norse Odin, and hence Woden in Britain. There is also the particular branch of Celtic Christianity that was of significant influence in these early centuries, in the way that Gnosticism was in the Middle East; I see a lot of interchange and creative fusion in these various processes.

What I think has happened is that we have allowed esoteric or mystical Christianity to be subsumed in a view of Christianity, the religion, that was progressively used as a political force and social means of control over the first millennium. This is what is extant and presented to us, but is not all that Christianity is, which Gnosticism – to me at least – more than adequately demonstrates. I have no truck with distancing myself from the Pauline version with its blatant patriarchy, misogyny, denial of the body (as a way of getting to control sexuality), and political ambition. But, to me, this is simply one branch (and a very limited one) of a trend of appreciating ourselves as paradoxically divine, or human-divine, which indigenous Heathen spirituality would recognise and embrace.

Medicine

I bring in comments about medicine for several reasons. Medicine is my trade and I was in formal medical practice for several decades as a holistic physician and medical psychotherapist. The runes initially revealed themselves to me in my exploration of my heritage and spiritual background to healing.

Documented Anglo-Saxon medicine occurs late in the first millennium, but it is imbued with Christian ritual in a way that demonstrates that the medicine of that era would also have been more ritualised generally; a lot of Christian interpolation in the texts can be easily differentiated to reveal other ritual input and belief systems. Woden, himself, is mentioned in the *Nine Herbs Charm* recorded in the tenth century *Lacnunga* manuscript, being a collection of miscellaneous Anglo-Saxon medical texts, written mainly in Old_English and Latin. *Lacnunga* is a rendering of the Modern English word, *Remedies*. The charm is intended for the treatment of poisoning and infection by a preparation of nine herbs. The ritual input is of a distinctly magical character. Over time, and from the end of the millennium, the medical system adopted in Britain became more Mediterranean, so reflecting the religious and language changes, including the written material and their scripts.

In most cultures, medicine is deeply integrated with the spiritual and social systems in which it is practised. In the western world, our scientific medicine is the exception to the rule. To use modern terminology, the medicine of the Heathen era was holistic. In fact, it is only in the last few hundred years that we have adopted a purely scientific, rational and technological approach to medicine. Most cultures have not, and even in the West there is a progressive reintegration of more holistic approaches, including those from other cultures and times. These trends indicate not simply a regression, but a retrieval of health and medical systems from the past that we have neglected in our headlong rush into scientific medicine, the limitations of which we are now beginning to fully appreciate.

This work is not about medicine. However, I want to draw attention to the way that medicine fits in the Anglo-Saxon world and evolved within it, as well as the similarities and overlap with language and religion. There is no doubt that, as a ritual technique used in magic and healing, the runes would have been an integral component of healing at the level of practice and delivery. It is this aspect of the runes that I employ in my own work, so I am aware of and experienced in their relevance and applicability, given that I take a magico-mystical perspective born of that era into the work I do and my life generally, yet in a modern context.

Magic

As with my comments with medicine; *Spellbinding* is not primarily a work about magic. But more than with medicine, the runes are involved with magic in a fundamental way. In the modern context, this is mainly in the area of divination, but is this the only way they were used? I don't think so, because divination is a receptive process of appealing to the psychic world beyond (a god, the gods, or supernatural forces) to give us information or to intercede on our behalf, somewhat like prayer. Magic is more than this; it is operative, where the practitioner actively participates in the process with the use of the will, or intent.

Magic routinely involves the use of words and language, which are used to access and channel magical power in accordance with the will, or ritual intent. In this respect, the use of language takes the non-verbal magical act or ritual to a different level, where the practitioner and participants are more emotionally involved in the process, be it ritualised or otherwise. It is also language, combined with the use of magical techniques including the runes, that sets humans apart and implies an active relationship with powers beyond, drawing them into the process. It is a co-operative relationship.

Words spoken in a specific context or framework are considered to have magical power; therefore, not all speech is magical. The language of magic is highly emotional by using words in a metaphoric and symbolic manner, so creating links between the unseen realities and their power to and in the mundane world. The use of magic is sacred, and the way the words are used – choice, phrases, and style – is what makes the use of language magical, lifting it above the profane.

We are familiar with these words and language in prayers and blessings, even if we are not routinely or emotionally connected with them; except in time of stress, fear, or need when they – seemingly paradoxically – become more effective. They can be used in chants, chanting, and in song, such as hymns. A spell or charm is the use of words or phrases that are considered to invoke a magical effect or outcome. Spells can summon a supernatural agent or being, including to prevent a person from taking some action, or compelling them to undertake one dictated by the spell, as governed by the practitioner. The line between good (white) and bad (black magic) is intuitively obvious here, so I will not further explore it.

In spells and charms the practitioner would value the inherent power within the words being used, as would the audience. Features such as acting, performance generally, as well as the ritual and ceremonial context are all important components. All these features combined make a powerful emotional mixture with potential psychic outcomes; a pattern well known to the practitioner and those who have experienced it. To the lay outsider, unless the emotional connection is activated (often demanding the suspension of existing belief systems), the effect will be disproportionately low, or absent. This inherent paradox is well understood by the practitioner, who would not routinely choose to persuade, but to demonstrate, if so inclined.

All the above is a brief and very condensed overview because, as stated, this is a book about the Futhorc, not magic and its practice; although I lie a little, as we will be going deeper into all this in the Spellbinding section that follows. But it can be immediately seen that the runes fulfil many of the functions of magical practice at the simple level of use of words, phrases, and language. However, the informed reader will note that potentially any language can fulfil this magical function, it is undertaken according to the above criteria. So, what makes runes any different?

It is because the runes have the words and phrases, as well as poetry, as part of the lexicon. They can be readily employed, if they *talk* to you, and you feel them to be part of your heritage and culture. If not, they probably won't work magically. Modern words and phrases can be used, but it requires a symbolic sensibility and a fair amount of creative innovation. It is something I am keen to do in my own ritual and ceremonial practice however, because it appeals to and involves others in ways that don't demand an undue suspension of judgement. With magic, it is different. Runes, to my mind, are a product of metaphysical or archetypal forces, so the shapes themselves contain power and magic.

To illustrate this, I will give you a window into practice using the runes. If I am counselling someone in difficulty, I may or may not know what this is in any detail, or even at all. I can ask the client to do a rune reading based on the problem, and then start to interpret it for them. By now, and in a combination of ways, I will have ascertained a lot further information, not only from the runes, but also from their demeanour, body language, and my psychic feeling about them. I can then use the reading as a means to convey my message; that is, the message the runes have given, as well as the collateral information I have gleaned.

I will try and use language that is intentional and meaningful, such as short phrases, words that I *know* have power; which are frequently Old English, by the way. I will perform and act to the part of the magician, with authority and conviction, yet I will remain open to the changing emotional and psychic landscape of the consultation. I may use this book to augment what I am conveying, to give a weight of authority and power. But at all times, I need to be aware of my client and where they are moving psychically, and not to exert my own judgements or preferences.

To those aware of the psychotherapeutic process, this is all familiar. But it is more ritualised and employs techniques that directly engage spirit. Dreams and their interpretation could be considered something similar. Combined, I find the use of a rune reading to go deeper and more quickly than other approaches; partly this is because the authority is not just invested in my personality, so the psychic territory can be traversed more readily and accurately. But, like any approach, it is a skill, and demands teaching and practice.

Yet this is not stage magic. I am not doing this to demonstrate power – even though I am actively using it – or to intentionally trick or otherwise manipulate my client. However, the tendency to misuse the power and come under the thrall of the Trickster can be great. Ultimately, there is a faith in the process beyond all judgement and that I, as practitioner, am a vehicle of the forces I invoke and share. My will is Thine. How I use these forces and information will obviously depend on my skill and the connection I have with my client.

Sexuality

Is sexuality the elephant in the room? It is a component, even if implicitly so, of the sections to date: spirituality, medicine, and magic. Earlier, I discussed sexuality along with spirituality and magic as components of the Futhorc, and as with them, would like to extend this discussion further. I have already done this by adding medicine to the mix, and will go further in the next section with a more detailed discussion of the Anglo-Saxon understanding of the Soul, extending from the preliminary remarks about this in the Anglo-Saxon Mentality. But the first comment I would like to make is how we view sexuality in the present, and how this is entwined with our views on gender.

We are remarkably confused about gender. We have assumed that the scientific worldview would provide us with clarity and that looking into the brain, such as the right hemisphere is masculine and the left is feminine, or the body and even genetics in more detail has not been rewarding. Next, we have gone to psychology and, Jung's attempts notwithstanding, we are still confused. How do I know all this? Because we still see gender in an oppositional way and we have become remarkably coy (call it 'political correctness') about discussing it in an open way, so that the dialogue cannot creatively progress.

I am going to put my hat in the ring and provide a remarkably simplistic view of gender and sexuality. I actually do think it is this obvious, but we fail to see the wood for the trees. So, here goes ... the physical level, that is our bodies, we are principally two genders, male and female (please take note of the words – male and female). Beyond this there is some blending, but generally not a lot, and the amount where there is genuine physical gender confusion is relatively small.

Now to the psychology. We are both (that is male and female, both) masculine and feminine. Now masculine and feminine are not physical genders that are prone to a bit of blending, on occasion, they are pure principles; or, as Jung would have it, archetypes. And, to repeat my point, both men and women have masculine and feminine principles in their psychological make-up. These vary in expression in development, over time, in response to circumstance, in the bedroom, etc. etc. And we do a damn good job of projecting what we are not acknowledging at the time into the world, and on other groups or people. Result: havoc. Now add sex to the mix: WW III.

Now a peak into the Heathen psyche, and specifically that of the period under inquiry in this work. There appears to be much less conflict between the genders, a clearer partition of roles, and a rewarding of ability based on that – ability and not gender. There appears to be acceptance of any confusion and blending, particularly in shamanism, where this seems associated with wounding and healing in a profound social and spiritual way. The people who negotiated these traumas and confusions became the shamans, magicians, and healers.

Am I being naïve, unrealistic? Well, look at Woden. He is the stereotypical shaman and displays all sorts of masculine, even hyper-masculine qualities. But he is also profoundly versed in Seith magic, the art of magic according to the feminine. So, although the northern peoples seem to display strong gender-based roles, they also seemed to acknowledge, accept, and embrace the areas of confusion and trauma that we have difficulty with. Were the sexually and gender confused in our society to look deep into their own trauma and wounding, I believe we would have far less of a problem in the world, because this is also the first step in healing.

So far, so good. You might have enjoyed my brief analysis here, but what has that got to do with the runes, you may ask? As the runes appear to be a spiritual coded system to deal with life that is fundamentally holistic and includes medicine, magic, and religion, then why wouldn't the Futhorc include sexuality? After all, the main ceremonial times of the Celtic and Anglo-Saxon peoples include seasonal celebrations based on birth, life and death; isn't sexuality an integral part of the life cycle? And, if it is – as it is – why has it been excluded?

In some ways, these are not difficult questions to answer, and I have done this to some extent already. The Church, by separating the individual from their body and sexuality, psychically divides him or her. Birth and death have been the province of religion as well, although in later years it has ceded this to medicine and the scientific worldview. Yet religion has kept ownership of sex, in spite of modern medicine and infectious disease. And the modern Church is essentially patriarchal, misogynist and erotically-denying. Sexuality is not seen in the context of the human life cycle, as it is in the agricultural and hunter gatherer peoples.

Yet this was not the case with Heathen peoples, either in history, or in contemporary equivalent cultures. Divide people from their sexuality by making them feel guilty about it, and then you control them. Rub it in by making emotion a second-rate psychic function and the populace is further disempowered. Don't let them have contact with birth or death either. Make warfare mechanised and brutal, so that the warrior and sacrifice are no longer honoured ... get the picture?

Now I do not think that the Futhorc contains a hidden sexual pathway or initiation process. The myths associated with the Heathen gods were overtly sexual, sometimes blatantly so, thus rendering any undue coding unnecessary. Instead, and as I have indicated at various points in the discussion of the individual runes, the sexual aspects are but one facet of the condensed symbolism that also includes nature, the seasonal cycles, wounding and trauma, warriorhood, magic, and social functions. Sexuality was not separated and is readily apparent in the first rune row of **Feoh**.

How this was expressed in such areas as ritual and ceremony, between the sexes within and without a marriage, is open to question. Our understanding of some of the ceremonies indicate that birth, sex, marriage and death were all honoured and deeply reflected in the cosmology and seasonal cycles. In the myths there are narratives of sex with animals and even with the land; what are we to make of these, apart from seeing them in a greater mythic and spiritual context? Is sex expressed in ritual and ceremonial formats? I believe it was, because I deduce that it must have been. And it is only our modern sensibilities and conditioning that would have difficulty with this.

To integrate all this into some deeper ritual context would require more work. Firstly, for us to strip away the accretions and prejudices we carrying from our conditioning, and secondly to have the tools to explore them. It is a work to be done, and is there for the doing. Obviously, some modern traditions, such as Wicca and various magical societies, have sought to do this; but it is by no means coherent and systematised in a way that is readily understandable, and therefore acceptable to modern society in general. One can only go so far with an intellectual and intuitive understanding of the Futhorc, but my realisation as a consequence is that not only are sexual patterns inherent in it, they are there to be ritually enacted.

A closing word on gender and death. As with sexuality, these concepts symbolically permeate the runes, and in differing combinations. The clear differentiation that modernity makes seems less significant in traditional cultures. Is there an inherent wisdom here that we have lost? Maybe a few points to illustrate may help. Although we can identify gender in the runes, it is by no means clear cut. Nor is sexuality, which is largely inferred. There is a blurring of boundaries, maybe exemplified by Woden – feminine, creative, playful – that may portray these issues in a way that resolves a lot of our current rational approach.

Also, death is close to the surface in some runes, particularly in the rune extension, as with **Ear**. Death would appear to be far more connected to life than in our times, as would the spectre of violence. There are various areas that do not come easily to us moderns, such as the relation of violence to sex, and both to death. Such relationships indicate levels of our human experience as in say, sacrifice, that we do not understand so readily. A lot of this have related to our hyper-individualised existence, somewhat distanced from the whole psyche that we experience, as well as the image of death as represented by Christianity; but maybe no more.

The Heathen worldview is quite different in degree and kind; there is much that we have lost touch with, which the runes remind us of and help in that holistic reconnection.

The Soul Complex

The *Soul Complex* provides a deeper and extended appreciation of the Anglo-Saxon Mentality presented earlier. It also forms a solid basis for the sections that follow. Having said this, it is about the soul specifically and only indirectly about the runes, as it was originally written as a separate paper. Although it takes the reader on a journey more specifically to understand and appreciate the Anglo-Saxon spiritual worldview, it is not essential reading in the continuity of *Spellbinding*. Should the reader desire to focus more specifically on the runes and runelore, little will be lost if this section is bypassed.

Introduction

A significant part of this section was covered earlier in the Anglo-Saxon Mentality, so there will inevitably be some overlap of that prior section: Treat any as revision and elaboration rather than duplication, as it is integral to furthering the discussion. It was considered necessary at that earlier prior point, so that the reader could gain some appreciation of the Anglo-Saxon mindset before engaging the runes. But there are meaningful extensions both ways from that prior limited outline of the soul complex: One way leads back to the physical body, and the other forward to the more transpersonal elements inclusive of the soul in the personal sense.

Therefore, this section is almost a topic in its own right and not fundamental in the context of the book as a whole. However, not only does it provide some sort of expansion and completion to the earlier Anglo-Saxon Mentality section, but it also opens the reader up to the rich continuum that can exist in a culture where spirituality is a more integral aspect of all aspects of life, and not marginalised or reduced to a rational and mechanistic psychology, as has occurred in the modern era.

The concepts of both soul and spirit are undergoing appreciable change and redefinition in the 21st century, as they emerge from the historical, religious, and cultural mists into the scientific era. An era that, in an attempt to either ignore these metaphysical entities or deny their existence, paradoxically seems to be led back to them at the extremes of any scientific discipline. Physics is probably the most notable in this regard, yet even psychology and medicine are following suit, even if reluctantly and belatedly.

Latterly, the breakdown of religious social organisation in the West; the attendant rise of science as a pseudo-religious *scientism*; the advent of the so-called New Age; the influx of eastern religions and their philosophies, and the retrieval of primitive and archaic perspectives all make for a heady mix. Added to this is the necessary appreciation of the educational, cultural, and ancestral background of any commentator (including me, here) and their prejudices, which demands the reader examine his or her own views in a similar manner to then arrive at their own conclusions and definitions.

In this section, I am offering some initial reflections on the subject of soul and spirit, their connection, and points of differentiation. These remarks serve as a starting point to undertake that necessary preliminary exercise of reflection prior to defining or redefining the soul with this traditional input; from there to briefly engage issues that lead on from this, such as soul loss and its retrieval within any healing approach.

Commonly, we see the body as the container for the soul, and in the same analogous way we can see the brain as a container for the mind. Or, if we see the soul connected with the body at all, we can tend to a more Christian position, where the soul is more intimately bound with spirit and even separate from the body. Both these latter restricted and simplistic viewpoints are drawn into question here.

The soul may be appreciated as a kind of middle ground between spirit and the physical body from the perspective of the perennial philosophy, such that it can readily be confused with the term, *mind*. The body, or body-mind, itself can be viewed as the physical representation, mirror, or expression of the soul. From this viewpoint, the soul is seen to include the body, but to extend beyond it in various non-physical, or metaphysical yet meaningful ways. However, these extensions are not to be seen as derived from the body, but more the other way around. In this worldview – which I endorse – the body is more a derivative or expression of the soul in physical space and material reality.

Using this understanding of body and soul as an analogy, the physical world might be seen as the equivalent external representation, mirror or reflection of the spirit. Here can be detected an initial differentiation of soul and spirit; that the soul is more representative of the individual, experienced directly and connected somehow to the physical body, whereas spirit is of a broader, impersonal, or transpersonal reality. In religious terminology, the soul is therefore more immanent and spirit transcendent; terms to which I will return. This immanence implies that the soul is a reflection of spirit within time.

The senses can be seen to mediate between the body – and hence the soul – and the external world, which itself reflects spirit. This all gives us an initial holistic perspective that precludes the body-mind duality of our modern era, both religiously and scientifically. Our restricted – and restrictive – cognitive viewpoints of dualism and reductionism demand expansion and inclusion of others, such as abstraction and also emotion, to become truly holistic.

These various extensions to and from the body that constitute the soul may be described in modern physical and psychological terms. They include the mind, emotions, and the individual will. Such supportive terms as focus, attention, and intent can be identified, as can the vexed but essential issue of power. We are accustomed to see these associated more with the body and specifically the brain, but they can also – and more appropriately – be seen to extend beyond it to the non-physical dimensions of the intellect and creative imagination, as well as broaching domains like morality and ethics. In general, it is a mistake to see the brain, which after all is simply an organ in the body, as equivalent to the mind, and hence the some scaled-down perspective of the soul.

These latter aspects can be seen to overlap and maybe connect with what we have formerly considered as the spiritual world, mainly because they have been the province of religion and its symbolic systems. The idea of soul can then become identified with or even subsumed by spirit, and hence seem to appear unattainable, as in the recent era. This points to another important factor: An individual soul that has developed a creative and symbolic capacity has a more autonomous access to the world of spirit. Other influences that impinge on the soul and connect with it, possibly originating more in the realm of spirit, include collective memory (that may comprise what I refer to as our *psychic DNA*) and hence our ancestral history.

Collectively, these views raise certain questions: Does the soul originate with the body or precede it? Or is it developed by the individual in their lifetime? Does the soul, with its character of a more immanent spirituality, transcend the physical lifetime and defeat death? Do we all have souls, and can they be lost and hence retrieved? Does the greater spiritual reality contain forces or powers that can supervene and invade and possess the soul, when it is vulnerable, as with pain and trauma?

An authentic understanding of spiritual reality may go some way toward appreciating and even answering such questions. From the comments above and as already discussed, the world of spirit may be seen as more transcendent (or *beyond*), in contrast to the more immanent (or *immediate*) soul. Spirit can be seen as being beyond three-dimensional space and time; although it would be a mistake to see it as simply infinite and eternal from a more concrete reality-bound perspective. There might be gradations between these extremes, which the concept of soul may encompass and include, and which figures such as elves, faeries or angels symbolise. In general, the world of spirit is mysterious and more visionary and mythic in quality when approached. It also appears to be autonomous, self-regulatory, readily leading to the idea that spirit – as *God* – is omniscient, omnipotent, and omnipresent (all knowing, powerful, and seeing).

The soul appreciates the world of spirit most readily through its higher intellectual, intuitive and imaginative functions, and identifies it within symbolic systems and in mythic forms. It is important not to confuse these images or forms, which the soul can more directly appreciate and express, with the ultimately mysterious reality itself that is probably beyond these representations. Qualities considered higher, such as beauty, goodness, and love, could be considered the province of spirit that can be apprehended and better appreciated by a developed and mature soul rather than simply the cognitive mind.

The term *higher* also points to our tendency to see spirit associated with the sky or heavens, and lends itself to envisage intervening and mediating forms, such as angels and the more modern notion of archetypes. In contrast, the soul is more characterised by *depth*, mistakenly identified in some religious systems as *fallen*. Depth implies the soul's recognition of death and the associated phenomena of trauma, wounding, and suffering; challenges that it must face in its reconnection (or ascent) to the world of spirit that is maybe a lifetime's task or work.

One way to retrieve the western soul would be through Christianity. To do this, I would take a route around the distortions and even negations that the soul has suffered under institutional Christianity over the centuries, and explore its understanding in such esoteric areas as Gnosticism. Traditions that engage the participant actively in the spiritual process, such as alchemy and magic, have had a predictably enigmatic relationship with the institutional Church.

Closer to home, I believe the Celtic Church probably contained a healthier perspective, stemming from the Heathen spiritual traditions that preceded it, and implied in the imagination with figures like the Druids. However, with the eclipse of the Celtic by the Roman Church, this is difficult to unearth. And, anyway, this perspective was contained in the Heathen traditions from which Christianity itself arose, and that continued for many centuries into the Christian era in Britain. There are signs they continue still, at least in memory and the folk traditions. There are several paths to and meanings of redemption herein, it would seem.

The Old English Body-Soul Complex

An Overview

In this section I am using the term *Old English* to describe the *Body-Soul Complex* as opposed to Anglo-Saxon, because a lot of material here is drawn from the language of the time and is the preferred term used by those who study this language period, with its progression into and contrast with *Modern English*. I further see it as inclusive of the Anglo-Saxon period, the Celtic that preceded it, as well as other less well-defined peoples and language groups. Elsewhere, I prefer the more descriptive term Anglo-Celtic to cover this period of time from pre-history to the end of the first millennium.

I call the Old English body-soul a complex, because it is both a *complex* of many facets and also complex in nature. As an aside: Were the body-mind 'problem' to be looked at in a similar manner and not in the dualistic way requiring some sort of unification, as it currently is, then we would get beyond some difficulties that modern western medicine, psychology and even philosophy are troubled by.

The body-soul is a more complicated entity than the single one implied within Christianity, which is unduly simplistic and serves to support the erroneous idea of human *perfection*. The Complex is a kind of consolidation of various parts that, under certain conditions, can separate from the unity and act autonomously. Some of these parts could even be seen as autonomously conscious, and lead to complex positions with respect to concepts such as *soul loss* and *spirit possession*.

The various facets of the soul that are related to each other are inclusive of the physical body and collectively comprise the Old English pre-Christian perspective. I trust the soul will be seen as a richer and more diverse concept than the limited one in Modern English, which pales into insignificance compared to other cultures, including the modern German one that has a far more nuanced view of the term soul.

Compare the Old English to the Christian spiritual perspective: The Church aggregates soul within spirit. The Pauline soul is primarily a spiritual element, identified with the godhead and therefore dichotomous to the physical self. Maybe this gives the only avenue of salvation as Jesus Christ: Could he thus be considered a symbol of the soul? As an image in this Christian view, the soul is left in the body as some sort of homunculus that departs it on death. Christianity today relates the soul to the afterlife, and not the body or mind in this life, except where sin is concerned. It might be worth bearing in mind that the philosopher Descartes, a devout Christian, considered that "some part of the brain served as a connector between the soul and the body and singled out the **pineal gland**." The Christian position could be considered incomplete, at best, and confused, at worst.

In contrast is the Heathen concept of the soul complex, which is both body-soul and spirit-soul (both in this life and beyond, encompassing wholeness and difference). It is the connecting bridge between the body and spirit, and somewhat analogous to the manner in which emotion connects or includes body and mind. The complex of body, emotion, and mind reflects the soul in the world; this is not simply a metaphor, in my view. Paracelsus' view that emotion is the vehicle of the soul may also be relevant here. A full appreciation of this concept, with its inherent subtleties and complexities, renders the modern body-mind dichotomy and duality as simplistic, reductionist, and materialistic – as well as largely irrelevant.

In what follows, I have taken a position that embraces the views of several commentators, and then amalgamated them with my own researches, deductions and conclusions, where appropriate. This inevitably extends to drawing upon associated cultures, particularly the Germanic and especially Old Norse (or ON), where these positions were more extant in the Anglo-Saxon period, due to the comparatively later significance and infiltration of Christianity in those countries. I have tried to enrich this further on occasion with some rather amateurish etymology, based more on psychological association than academic accuracy.

I find it interesting that Old Norse had no distinct concept of the soul prior to Christianity, indicating that this may have been the case with the Heathen Anglo-Saxons. This does not negate its existence, although Christianity might see it this way. Instead, the term *Soul* could have been adopted to unify disparate parts of the individual, which the Heathen may already have seen as united or whole in a *holistic* manner; that is, more than the sum of the parts. It may be that the Old English term for the soul, *Sawol*, or *Sal*, is a consequence of Christianisation, as it is not found as a distinct entity elsewhere. *Sawol*, is also a feminine noun, which is of interest with what is to follow.

Body-Mind

For an initial orientation toward the Old English (or OE) appreciation of the soul, I am taking the modern sensibility of body and mind as a skeletal framework, without recourse to the less well-known and appreciated elements, which will follow in the next section. I think such an approach prepares for these less well-known elements and concepts, although they may become more familiar in the reading, particularly if this ancient world is part of one's personal heritage.

In Old English, the physical body is called the *Lic (n)*, which also relates to a corpse; that is, a body without the other animating elements with which it is associated, when alive. It is believed that it is the gods who provide appearance, movement, and strength; that is, animate and even populate the body. Specifically, the breath of life is considered a gift of the god Woden (see *Wod*, to follow) that links the body and soul. I came across an interesting metaphor in my research, that "the genes serve as the warp that shapes the weave", which feels an apt description of the association of the non-physical forces with the otherwise inert physical body. It also demands we look at DNA in a more limited manner; both less mechanically and also with less importance than we currently do, I would suggest.

Hyd (f) is an Old English precursor to our modern term *hide* and its multifarious meanings, and *Scinn (n)* to the actual skin. *Hyd* indicates the shape of the body; an ethereal image of the energy matrix within which the body – *lic* – is held. The *hyd* is another intermediary between the physical and spiritual, and also contains other mental elements to be described. It is considered to protect the forming soul prior to birth, as well as guiding and shaping the body, or *lic*, in its formation. As such, the *hyd* can be considered the skin of the soul, inclusive of, but not merely that of the body, which is the *scinn*. It may be that the *Hyd* can inhabit the body after death and be a more immediate form ancestor worship with access to the accumulated knowledge of the deceased. It could also explain the phenomenon of ghosts.

The broader concept of mind is more easily – at least initially – divided into three relatively familiar sections that connect with the body, with an additional fourth feature that is less well appreciated.

The concept, thought, is called *Hyge (m)*, which is the reasoning born of information gathering and memory retrieval. Essentially it is our cognitive selves which, when combined with *Mynd* (below) becomes intelligence. This function is closely related to perception and hence the senses, as well as intention or will. It appears to be the basis of personality, as we understand it in modernity. What is of interest is that the deliberate manipulation of the *hyge* with the *hyd* is considered the basis of magic, particularly shamanic journeying. However, if strong enough, the *hyge* may be powerful enough to influence others without recourse to other mental or soul entities.

From a physical perspective *hyge* would seem to relate to the left cerebral hemisphere of the brain. The rational and logical left hemisphere is considered masculine in the modern era, at least colloquially. And, interestingly, *hyge* is a masculine noun in Old English. There are also (maybe) some frontal lobe functions implied, as well. In fact, the Old English mental worldview generally maps well onto the brain, and would be an interesting route of further study.

A shamanic practitioner takes on the *hyd* in an animal form for travelling away from the body as the *hyge*. In this respect, there is an equivalence to modern idea of astral travelling, although the journeying the practitioner undertakes is commonly in animal form, maybe in the form of the shamanic *power animal*. It is stressed that this process is not simply within the imagination, but is also considered literal within Heathen culture. There are also associations here with magical *shape-shifting*, death, and the phenomena of ghosts and spectres.

Mynd (f) is memory of a personal nature accumulated in the present lifetime, resulting in learned knowledge and wisdom. However, it is related to a further dimension, sometimes called *Urthanc* (*Ur*, or primitive 'thought'), which is inborn and related to ancestral memory. This may relate to Jung's Collective Unconscious, racial memory, or the tribal mind. In other words, it is thought that is inborn and considered closely related to the physical instincts. This latter collective aspect is considered to separate from the body at birth, leaving a varied component in the soul. Neuro-physiologically, *mynd* relates to the right cerebral hemisphere, and the instincts to the more primitive brain and body, generally. *Mynd* is feminine, as the right hemisphere is often considered to be.

Mod (n) is emotion and the related mood. (Here, as elsewhere, the close association of the Old English words with Modern English is notable). Associated with the neurophysiological limbic system, *mod* occupies a central and possibly unifying function in the Old English mental economy. Functionally, *mod* relates more to *mynd* than *hyge*, and this also appears the case neuro-physiologically. It is considered the metaphoric heart and, of interest, the Old English view was that what we now recognise as the mind resided in the chest; maybe this is a reference to rational feelings. We do know that there are significant connections between the brain and the heart. As elsewhere, we may have lost much wisdom in our overemphasis of the brain.

Along with the instinctual part of the mind, *mod* is connected to the *lic* through the nervous and hormonal systems. With the intellect – maybe the combined *hyge* and *mynd* – *mod* may comprise the individual's psychic reality and even transport him or her beyond objective-subjective dualism. Although conjecture, it does indicate the unifying and connecting function with which people of the time saw *mod*.

Why I believe *mod* is important, beyond its comparative negation in the West in the modern era, is that its stimulation through shamanic techniques, such as ritual drumming and dancing, leads to a connection with the *Wod*, or ecstasy. This is the domain of creativity and the imagination, of ecstasy and divine madness (think Bacchus or Dionysus), which is stimulated and expressed when in harmony with the other mental functions, as driven via the *mod*. This is not simply conjecture, as modern evidence is beginning to support this viewpoint. If disordered, as with overstimulation or the injudicious use of hallucinogenic drugs, then insanity can result, thus offering an alternative view of psychosis and (maybe) its potential management.

Where is the *wod* located? It may well be the pineal gland that Descartes saw as the seat of the soul. It is interesting that the powerful hallucinogen, dimethyl tryptamine (DMT), is also found in the pineal gland. *Wod* is, of course, related to the god Woden, who had many shamanic and magical functions that permeate all of those facets described here. Some see this as the *daimon* or *genius*; I see it as the connecting point of the unified soul with the transpersonal spiritual reality beyond, maybe the *nous* of Christianity. In Old English, the *wod* could be seen as the soul's home prior to physical existence. It is possibly here that the personal will can be seen to be directed by thoughts (*hyge*) and feeling (*mynd*), guided by passion (*wod*), and driven by emotion (*mod*).

Beyond the Body-Mind

Extending from the body are two further closely related elements that also have animal association, though distinct from the *hyd*. *Luck*, maybe the 'Guardian Spirit', is a source of personal power. In the body this can relate to bodily heat and the blood. It is connected to the family soul and hence more transpersonal in nature, although in the *weave* it may be seen metaphorically as genetic influences. Its image may be that of the individual themselves.

The *Fetch* or *Familiar* is a guardian, though more a wanderer (interestingly, one of Woden's characteristics). It may have an animal or geometric form, but is commonly a female human. The Fetch travels and brings back information and insight, through intuition; it thus has shamanic and magical characteristics. Some commentators consider the Fetch to be of the opposite sex to the physical body; however, I tend to consider it – her – feminine for both sexes. So, it is also closely related to the ON *fylgja*. In contrast to *luck*, the *familiar* seems to be more personally related to the individual. *Luck* may be a more recent word, not distinctly or particularly Old English. It is considered a transpersonal ancestral force that is sometimes personified, usually as a female form, or takes animal shape.

It might assist to describe the ON *fylgja* in its own terms; that is, Old Norse, and to dip into it more generally for comparison. This may help shed further light on the OE terms, *fetch*, *familiar* and *luck*. *Fylgja* is a guardian spirit or guide. It can be an animal, abstract or geometric form, or a person of the opposite, or female sex. It has a nature and form similar to its owner, so can reflect the *hyge* and *hyd*, respectively. Although of an animal nature, *fylgja* is often a female figure, with resonances here to Jung's concept of anima. It is therefore also closely related to the modern concept of soul. The *fylgja* is considered to be a spirit that carries fortune for the individual, as well as being connected to their fate or *wyrd*. It can also be community-based or tribal, as in totems, and be passed in the bloodline; something shamanism recognises in its practitioners.

The *fylgja* leaves its possessor at death and becomes an independent being; it is not synonymous with the Christian concept of soul. It can also transfer to another family member. When I start to look at the *fylgja* this way, it starts to make intuitive sense to me and fills a void in an otherwise personalistic and rational psychology of modern times. Not only does it unite the feminine side of my own nature, but I suspect it does this for both men and women, as the *fylgja* fulfils a bridging function between our material and spiritual worlds.

But this is not simply confined to the term *fylgja*, it also relates to concepts like the *Norns* and *Valkyries*, which I will describe shortly. More significantly, this whole field of the feminine describes the magical branch of *Seidr* (*Seith* in OE), which is closely involved with the shape-shifting and mental projection already described, but takes them to a deeper and more spiritual level. In some ways, maybe a development of shamanic practice, *Seidr* indicates that the power of the feminine was a respected and integral part of Old Norse magical practice, and hence Heathen practices more generally, including the Anglo-Saxon.

The related ON term, *hamingja*, closely overlaps these concepts, but may indicate the force of *luck* itself and be the transpersonal ancestral component of these overlapping terms. Some of this confusion in terms may relate to distinguishing the energy or force from its image, in my opinion, and warrants further inquiry. I, like others, am also taking recourse to Old

Norse to try to obtain clarity. Although close to Old English, they are not exactly synonymous and, on occasion, can obfuscate as much as clarify. There are degrees of subtlety in these relationships and interconnections that we have yet to unearth, separate from our customary rational way of appreciating them.

Hamingja is the total amount of power that a person is in possession of, influencing wealth and success (some similarity to *luck* exists here). It is closely related to *fylgja*. My personal impression is that *hamingja* includes not only *fylgja* but also the mental functions (*hyd* and *hyge* in OE) to express it. There are many connections here with shamanic practice generally, and ON *Seidr* or OE *Seith* more specifically, such that the magical power resides in the feminine, as well as an animal or geometric shape; a symbol of power. Intuitively, there is a kind of masculine and feminine balance of magical forces here, with the masculine reliant on the feminine, although important in its expression, as ON *Galdr*.

Other terms, such as *Mægen* (spiritual power or strength), or *Orlog* (luck or fate), and *Wyrd* (fate or destiny) are also more Germanic and Nordic; although *wyrd* persists even into Modern English as *weird*. *Mægen* is connected to sacrifice; that is, the transfer of power to the gods in return for one's own empowerment. There are distinct connections here to ritual and ceremony.

Ond is an ON term for spirit or breath, and could be considered the *divine spark*, connected to reality and the power of place. *Ond* opens up the power of the voice, or *Galdr* (*Galdor* in OE) in magical terminology. It is connected to inspiration, ecstasy and hence the ON *Od*, the basis of the shamanic god Odin, and hence to the OE *wod*, discussed earlier. Old Norse terms they may be, but their lack or tenuous connection in Old English does not imply their absence, simply that they are inferred but not clearly identified.

It is to be remembered that we are exploring an era in English history, the Anglo-Saxon period of 412 – 1066 AD, where the Christian influence was already present and becoming increasingly dominant at the beginning of the European migrations, such that by the middle of this period England was more formally Christian. In contrast, during this whole period Scandinavia was generally free of Christian influence, becoming Christianised at around the same time the Anglo-Saxon era finished in England. The effect of this existing influence on the peoples who brought their heathen beliefs to England would have been significant, so obscuring much depth and wisdom. To my mind, the actual term soul itself is a significant case in point. Also, all written material was in the hands of the Church during this same period.

In addition to the above factors, the overlapping nature of our modern interpretations may indicate our lack of appreciation of the complexity and subtlety within and implied by these terms, rather than seeing them as being confused. Certainly, my exploration of them feels a work in progress, as I grapple with understanding them retrospectively from a modern position, as well as appreciating their meaning and significance in Anglo-Saxon times. The reason Germanic, Nordic, and sometimes Icelandic languages are drawn upon for understanding is that the Christian influence was far later there.

Whilst their complexity has been relatively lost in Modern English, we can draw on these other traditions to indicate the depth and richness in the individual's complexity. There was considerable overlap in the English, Germanic, and Scandinavian traditions, after all. That these terms indicate such issues as fortune being inherited and/or fated, as well as the close relationship to animal or spiritual figures (often feminine), indicates avenues into the transpersonal domains – and their influence on the individual – that lend to further exploration. There is much here that is encouraging.

There is a plethora of further overlapping terms; such as the already mentioned *Sawol (f)*, often considered the soul after death, and therefore related to the Christian soul. By contrast *Feorh (m)* is the principle of life and is often seen as synonymous with the Old English soul itself, as an animated body. Although many of these terms are non-physical, they have an intimate relationship with the body, as recognised in the images of animals and people. Whilst distinct from the more mental features, there are obviously several points of resonance between the various elements that may be detected. Also, the deep connection with fauna and hence nature, and the world, is not to be ignored.

My initial impression of the terminology is that there was and is much duplication: Maybe this has been brought about by overlapping languages; differing belief systems; the influence of Christianity; the tyranny of time and of history. But the more I have explored these terms, the more subtle and differentiated I have found them to be. It is simply that they do not fit into our modern intellectual and linear straightjackets, such as the 'body, mind/soul and spirit' of perennial philosophy. In fact, this research has caused me to reject such simplicity in favour of this ancestral subtlety and wisdom. I am also impressed how this worldview forges into parapsychological realms in a way that we lose with our modern rational, reductive, and scientific viewpoint of such phenomena. We have lost much, it seems.

There are other facets that connect, but maybe take us too far beyond the soul complex. *Wyrd* has been mentioned, which we recognise as fate or destiny in the modern era, and which may relate to the *fetch*. There are also various other images of a feminine nature, such as the Old Norse *Norns* (the weavers of fate) and the *Valkyries* (conveyors of the soul to the afterlife), who serve domains like *wyrd*, or have a more spiritual function, being closely related to the gods. Maybe this takes us into Old English mythology and too far afield, but I do find the feminine imagery significant in what was thought to be a predominantly masculine culture, as intermediaries between the gods the individual, and more. In an era blighted with sexual and gender controversy, the enigmatic and shamanic figure of Woden, at one level so hyper-masculine, yet containing many inherent levels of gender ambiguity (particularly in the magical realms), may have much to inform us.

In conclusion to this section, one issue to highlight is the apparent dichotomy between imagination and reality, as well as the more modern subjective-objective duality. Imagination permeates the soul complex, and is a vital ingredient in shamanic and magical practice. I think it is fair to say that Old English does both suffer these contrasts to the point of dichotomy and opposition, but appreciates them in a more creative manner. The imagination may help to mobilise the *hyge* in animal form to depart the body, but maybe it is also literally true; that the traveller becomes the animal, and leaves his or her body in a trance state whilst journeying. My personal impression is that this attitude is one that serves much in the way of exploration of tradition, and that our modern scientific, reductive, and quantitative cognitive approaches do not appreciate the full picture. One needs to enter into the mentality of the time, I believe, to fully appreciate what is happening.

Reflections

I think most readers will have followed my exegesis up to the Beyond the Body-Mind section (above), because of the familiarity with modern concepts in various disciplines, such as neuroscience and academic psychology, but then found that the territory became much more unstructured and fluid. Some commentators have tried to impose some sort of structure here, but as you may have experienced in reading that section, this can be frustrating, confusing and – in my view – inappropriate. Instead, rather like an archaeological dig, we are left with bits and pieces, fragments of a past that may have been more unified then. Bringing them together into some sort of holistic unity is as much an art as a science.

Or maybe this is not the way to proceed in this inquiry. Maybe consciousness was not as individualised then as we see it presently. And maybe collapsing all these concepts and ideas into an individualistic framework is destined to fail, unless we entertain some kind of transpersonal and spiritual perspective. My personal orientation, inferred in preceding comments, is that Christianity, as a political and social religious force, has done much to repress the Heathen heritage it subsumed. I have found this leaves us with a contemporary vision of the soul that is distant, incomplete, and confused with the term spirit, and hence spirituality more generally.

I have taken pains to try and tease out the individual and personal aspects, because they support my interests, up to and including using this wisdom as a therapeutic and healing tool. In so doing, I have found that a shamanistic worldview, in its broad and not academically restricted sense, provides a framework for both the individual and transpersonal elements of the body-soul complex. Similarly, I think that Jung's explorations – not forgetting that Jung was a German-Swizz – are a similarly useful mapping process for much of the above.

In so many ways I find the basic and more individualistic structure of the Old English body-soul complex appealing. Whilst I am fascinated by the overlap of the more transpersonal aspects, with such areas as shamanism and Jungian psychology, I think there is a place for consolidating the personal and individual aspects of the body-soul complex away from our current dualistic, or body-mind viewpoint. I further think this matches our more modern, individualistic, and personal approach to consciousness, its role in healing, and furthers it in ways that our current materialistic, scientific, and reductive approaches cannot.

Simply put, this is because the Old English viewpoint provides a subtle, yet significant perspective: It sees that the individual body – including the brain – is somehow *distilled* from a vaster non-materialistic reality. However, it contains important and necessary connections with that reality for its very existence, and honours it – and its superiority – accordingly. But this does not ignore our individualised worldview, it simply sees it as a part of this greater continuum, and that there are demands and responsibilities that we can only meet from this individual perspective.

To my mind, this makes us co-creators in our health and wellbeing. There are significant responsibilities that stem from this position in modernity; such as being involved in our own healing journey, and that our narrative is important – even essential – to this process. The materialistic rush to quantify and normalise our health takes away this position and its responsibility. In our various modern medicinal systems, we are driven by protocols and statistics; the individual has become lost. It is not a surprise to me that, beyond such areas as accident and emergency, modern western medicine is severely wanting. And I am proposing that the body-mind complex of a bygone era may hold important clues in our journey of healing and its – synonymous – spiritual development.

Further and unstated, we are a long way, it seems, from fully appreciating all this material in a purely energetic manner, as it terms like vibration, rhythm, pulse, wave and resonance, even breath. This is certainly so in my fields of medicine and psychology, where any true healing perspective must necessarily include them. My impression is that this perspective, drawn from modern physics and even philosophy, may shine a much greater and more comprehensive light and render the term *complex* redundant.

The Body-Soul Complex in Modernity

In a way, I have taken the position of the perennial philosophy, and given the soul a position between the physical body, cognitive mind, and the metaphysical realm of spirit. In this, I have already adapted somewhat to modernity, although the picture I have built up of the Old English soul largely fits this scheme. I have made comment above, with reference to Jung and shamanism, that whilst the transpersonal (or *beyond* the personal), metaphysical (*beyond* the physical), and suprasensible (*beyond* the senses) realms are subjects in their own right, they are only touched upon in this discussion. However, the Anglo-Saxon Mentality and my analysis of the Old English body-soul complex naturally includes them in a more comprehensive manner.

Another significant point, or conclusion, drawn from the Old English material, is that the dynamic or energetic direction of flow, or power, is from above down – from the spiritual to the physical. In modernity, aided by materialistic science, we labour under the belief that the flow is the other way around, where it may well be better understood, but only in this modern restricted and rational worldview. Whilst emphasis on the spiritual and abrogation of personal control may define the Old English worldview from the modern perspective, it is my considered opinion that the pendulum has not only swung, but too much the other way. We have developed an arrogant positioning in our materialism, as well as an assumption about will, power, and control that I believe is largely erroneous.

Also, this may stand behind the rather trivialised term, *mind over matter*, implying that it is our thoughts that determine outcome. There is a vast amount of anecdotal and indirect evidence in medicine that this is the case in disease causation. But I think the term suffers from the fact that we are looking at thought in a limited and overly cognitive way. It also implies the equation that the mind is comprised of only our cognitive mechanisms, an assumption I hope I have done enough to dispel by now: The mind is far greater than mere thoughts, particularly if and when it conceptually approximates the soul.

The Personal Soul

I will be using this term to distinguish and integrate either all or selected aspects of the *lic, hyd, hyge, mynd, mod* and *wod* specifically; inasmuch as that is possible, given some of my preceding remarks! Alternatively, this Personal Soul could be called the Body-Soul, as the mental aspects have distinct physical correlations through the organ of the brain in modernity, as well as, in my opinion, the heart.

The *lic* is the body, enclosed by the *scinn*, and closely surrounded – enshrouded – by the *hyd*. This body is thus encased in an energetic matrix of a kind that may be referred to as etheric, and hence the now familiar term *etheric body*. Whilst this may be seen as the aura, it is not confined to humans, as indicated by Kirlian photography of plants and Sheldrake's morphic fields. It may also go a way to explaining issues like the phantom limb. To people sensitive to this etheric body, it may give an indication or otherwise of the health of the physical body, by such indices as colours perceived by the sensitive viewer. Such an attribute also implies a certain level of spiritual development in the viewer, although this need not always be the case.

The *hyge, mynd,* and *mod*, comprise a contemporary notion of the mind, as indicated earlier. That we often restrict this to the (masculine) *hyge* is unfortunate, because this constricts and limits the way we view not only other facets of the mind, or soul, but the transpersonal elements that impinge on them more readily, as with the feminine *mynd*. Maybe this is why the modern mind, that I am associating with the *hyge*, needs stimulation to create a different – altered – state of consciousness to escape its routine reality-bound basis. It may need the help of other facets, such as the *hyd* in animal, or other imaginary or symbolic form, to assist this process.

The *mynd* is less familiar; do not be mistaken by the phonetic sound! It seems to relate to memory beyond the cognitive, even racial (a view of *past lives*, possibly), and our creativity. The quality of feeling and the use of imagination may relate to the *mynd*, such that when the *hyd* travels in other realities, it may be through this portal, or with these attributes. As I have indicated, as the *hyge* may relate to the left cerebral hemisphere, the *mynd* may relate to the right. The frontal lobes, and other so-called executive functions, would also be involved.

It would be a mistake, in my view, to see this development of the central nervous system as recent and as the result of some sort of Darwinian evolutionary initiative. I am more inclined to see brain development to be the consequence of higher functions acting on, influencing, and stimulating the physical brain. (This might also relate back to earlier comments about mind over matter.) I see a similar mechanism to account for the development of speech. The idea that speech is the consequence of simple laryngeal development, as a consequence of natural selection, just doesn't make sense to me. Nor does the development of an opposable thumb, for that matter.

Yet the *hyge* and *mynd* alone may account for the idea of the intellect, but are not sufficient in themselves to account for a holistic mind, or supervening personal soul. The *mod* would seem to power and even direct these functions; after all, sexuality is used as a mechanism to stimulate consciousness in many – if not most – spiritual systems. Further, this is the basis of the passion and inspiration of the related *wod*, which may be a more direct connection to the gods and the spiritual world. I see the *mod* to occupy the emotional basis of the brain, related to our instincts and drives, and to be what we have in common with the animal kingdom. Its maturity may be essential for us to relate to and connect with animals, both for survival, but also for the altered states of consciousness the healer or shaman enters into.

That other spiritual facets have seen some sort of higher significance in the pineal gland has not escaped my attention. That the chemical DMT that is also found there, and common with many plants, hasn't either. DMT is one of the most, if not the most powerful psychedelic available on earth, and is the foundation of widespread shamanic usage, including healing and communal ceremony. *Wod* may have a home here, physiologically, and – as indicated earlier – the connection of the *mod* to the *wod* may be essential to shamanic healing rituals and achieving altered states of consciousness.

My personal impression is that this outline provides a fuller description of the mind, or the integrated 'I' of individuality, and one that is more holistic. I see that as being the *sawol, feorh*, or soul, in its more personal form. As it stands, it is very much a reflective unit within the present, but with extensions beyond. Without going into further detail here, I feel there are avenues of potential research and academic inquiry that could be explored.

The Liminal Soul

I am drawn here to the transpersonal and feminine dimensions of the *mynd*, as a contrast to the more masculine, or at least neuter tone of the above. The clarity of the previous section, and the readier application to modernity, start to drift a little here. There is also a lot that I am going to postpone to the next section, because I want to provide a clarity to this *in between* position, not overly influenced by more mythic and spiritual claims on it.

The feminine tone I find significant. I feel that this is a marginal, or *liminal* space – a portal between the worlds. The *mynd* seems both personal and transpersonal. Memory can be of this lifetime, but also ancestral, racial, or even mythic and archetypal, in the Jungian sense. The feminine is personal and a complement to the masculine facets to date, but also mythic and transpersonal. I believe the Jungian concept of *anima* relates to this state and place.

However, there is a subtle differentiation. The feminine images that extend from here have a more personal quality, unlike the more archetypal and goddess-like figures we will encounter. In a psychological sense this may represent personal images of the feminine that extend, via the mother, to ancestral and related others. It is of interest to me that magical and shamanistic lines of transmission often run in family lines.

I also believe it relates to something quite enigmatic in the northern traditions, and as exemplified by *Woden*; or, more clearly, ON *Odin*. The hyper-masculine figure that is Odin, is deeply connected to the feminine, either as his wife, Frigga, or more magically by the seeress, Freyja. It was Freyja that taught Odin the magic of *Seidr*, the *seething* magic of Old England. Although a wordsmith and a master of both the runes and *Galdr* (word magic, as in chants, charms, and spells), Odin needed to learn and practice *Seidr*. This rendered him ambivalent from a gender perspective, a position with alchemical overtones of higher evolution.

In my experience, Jungian psychology has reinstated this general position with the term, *anima*, and provided a more authentic view of *psyche* (the Greek word for soul) to psychology; a situation long overdue. But I think it could go further, were the more magical elements to be included. The shunning of magic because of its potential darkness, as implied in the figure of the sorcerer, is somewhat of an irony, as Jung himself was a fervent explorer of these nefarious realms of the human soul. Mind you, modern revivalism of many Heathen perspectives also finds this territory difficult to negotiate and, in my experience, lends itself to much social and political judgement.

This Liminal Soul has more psychic and hence parapsychological qualities, in the sense of having magical associations (through the feminine magical arts of *Seidr*), artistic (the *muse*), divinatory and parapsychological (*witch*) implications. It is deeply reflective and inter-related. As the earlier soul may have associations to what is known as the etheric body, this may be the astral body of spiritual terminology.

The Transpersonal Soul

This Soul is more a Spirit-Soul. But, unlike the Christian model of a soul that is transcendent, this retains its immanency. Via the *wod* or the god Woden/Odin, it has a deep connection in the physical body. I have referred to the association with the pineal gland so, in spite of its elevated position, even this soul is also associated with the body. Indeed, it would seem that this thread of connection is vital to human existence, and *wod* also implies 'inspiration', as in the breath. Also, in eastern spirituality, the pineal gland is considered the highest and most spiritual of the psycho-physical chakras; being the seventh, or crown chakra.

Of further interest here, is that there are some deep and significant resonances between eastern and specifically Indian spirituality, with what we are exploring here. There is also a common root of racial evolution in language and people, being known as Indo-European. Maybe these connections are not as far-fetched as they may seem, and it is valid to draw on the extant spirituality of the East, when that in the West has been – to my mind – quite severely disrupted from the time we are considering forwards. However, it is a case of drawing on, but not identifying with eastern systems; they may help re-establish our own blighted connections, but ultimately our heritage and ancestry may be western, not eastern. It is this we should be working with, hence the tone of this discussion.

In this realm, the feminine images are more transpersonal and archetypal, if we consider the *Valkyries, Norns,* and other figures of myth. In contrast to the figures in the liminal world of soul, they may be more objective than subjective; but does this make them 'real'? Here we are on delicate ground. Even the Jungian implication is that the soul and archetypes have an image, imaginary, or imaginative representation, implying that they are psychic products, but not real in the material sense. With this conclusion, I have no argument, but to say psychic material is not real in and of itself, is quite another matter; it most certainly is in the altered or ecstatic state. We could get into circular arguments here, joining Ufology and parapsychological ghost-hunters. Suffice it to say, I believe these images represent a psychic reality that is objective and available to people with sufficient psychic and spiritual development.

But what does all this have to do with the soul? When someone is sick or diseased, a medicine man or shaman may diagnose a *soul loss*. The treatment is for the shaman, in an altered state of consciousness (induced by various means), to *retrieve* the lost soul in the world of spirit, gods and goddesses, or other spectres – specifically in the underworld – and restore it to the sufferer. This is also the basis of modern psychotherapy, except that the therapist helps develop the skills of the client to retrieve their own soul, with his or her assistance. Further, this is a kind of metaphor for the difference in the individualisation of consciousness over nearly two thousand years, at the very least.

It may be that the therapist broadens and develops the skills beyond the mere cognitive *hyge* to enable it to be more flexible, by utilising other cognitive functions. From there to develop the feeling function of the *mynd*, as well as its creativity, imaginative, and intellectual abilities. And from there to become more conscious of the drives, instincts, and emotional life more generally, as with the *mod*. From this more unified and holistic perspective to be able to move to the liminal state of reflection, contemplation, meditation… and beyond. The client may find their more transpersonal soul – their vocation, fate, or calling – in the world of archetypes and gods. Or they, or more likely the therapist, may discover that they have been driven by one of them for its own purpose, as in *spirit possession*. Then, it is a question of removing this influence – *exorcising* – before moving forward. Good psychotherapy can achieve this, particularly with the inclusion of the transpersonal dimension and a shamanic temperament.

Yet we are not simply talking here of mental disturbance, such as anxiety or depression, or even psychotic states that bear a resemblance to spirit possession. We are also talking about the manner in which disruptions to the soul, caused by trauma as in mental illness, can also lead to sickness, disease and even death. There are echoes of these dynamics in much that enters the modern medicine consulting room. It is vaguely recognised by modern practitioners, particularly with the progress of experience; unfortunately, they lack the tools to be able to manage these problems beyond the physical. Even psychiatry is fundamentally materialistic in its pursuit of treatment.

The Integrated Soul

Writing the above section created two impulses: To try and unify these overlapping deductions and conclusions, and to honour modernity and other disciplines in the process. This will inevitably have some inherent limitations, but it may make the process and understanding clearer. There are inevitable lines of inquiry that extend from this brief review, which are either left for individual pursuit, or explored elsewhere.

The *personal soul* can be considered an aggregate of its own. Many commentators in the psychological and spiritual fields posit a triad of thought, feeling, and will in understanding an integrated 'I', as maybe *ego* or *self*. My understanding is that the personal soul, outlined above, represents this position and is a subtle fluid step beyond the more materially structured *self*, a step from space into time, perhaps?

The *liminal soul* is a portal of sorts. If the above is etheric, this is astral in nature, fluid and white. There is a deep feminine quality here, resonating with what is known as the *lesser work* in alchemy, and Jung's anima. In my opinion, there is a personal, familial, or ancestral flavour to any imagery encountered here, one that resonates with concepts such as *fetch* and *familiar*.

The *transpersonal soul* is possibly the step the individual takes through the doorway into the realm of spirit. It is the world into which the shaman steps and is the *greater work* of alchemy, marked by fire and red. There are many outlines to this in our culture, most notably the crucifixion and resurrection motif, where the importance of sacrifice is essential to the transition process. The role of suffering, and its representation in trauma and disease, has yet to be fully evaluated and integrated in modernity.

Yet this is also present in northern traditions in the figure of Woden and his self-sacrifice, like Jesus, on the 'Tree of Life' of the crucifixion. In fact, both figures are more god-men than mere portals or gods, they represent the stages the soul takes in its spiritual evolution. That Woden has a complex relationship with culture reinforces this; he is also seen as shamanic, and appealed to in the genealogy of Mediaeval English kings. Maybe this is most highlighted in the Arthurian corpus, where Merlin acts as a mediaeval Woden, and which moves to the Grail Corpus and its rich symbolism of spiritual development.

Conclusions and Relevance to the Runes

We are used to seeing alternative spiritual models in the current era. However, many of these are derived from other cultures and may not suit our cultural disposition and heritage. They may also be applied in a formulaic and mechanical way, appealing to the rational mind – the *hyge* – but little else; particularly when the distress and suffering may reside at the level of the soul, where the trauma has caused disruption in the psycho-physical unity.

It is my belief that the understanding of the Old English soul helps in this endeavour. Existing prior to Christianisation, it does not suffer the sort of traumas that this religion itself has perpetuated in the name of salvation, leading instead to a disruption of the soul and the sequelae I have described. There is much we need to overcome here at the social and religious level, and I feel that a more comprehensive understanding and nurturing of the authentic soul of our ancestry and heritage will assist in this endeavour.

If nothing else, I trust this exploration of the soul has opened the reader's mind not only to the Anglo-Saxon mindset, but also to its richness. In fact, one that may be more diverse and complex than the rather simple one we have inherited from science or the Church; that is, the soul equates to the mind (if you are of a rational and scientific disposition), or the soul is subsumed by spirit (if religious).

In fact, from an esoteric perspective, the Old English soul perspective appears to me to be more distinctly Gnostic from the modern viewpoint; which is a position that may yet emerge to bridge and reconcile the differences between science and religion. This makes me wonder whether this more Heathen and esoterically Christian position generally, and the runes in particular, might have a part to play in such a reconciliation and our present potential of psychic evolution; because we are most certainly in an era of great transition.

We seem to have gone down a long path away from the runes, or have we? One limitation of our understanding and usage of the runes in the modern era is that we do this with a modern mentality. So, it seemed relevant to me to explore the Anglo-Saxon Mentality as a way of giving the runes context and providing the reader with a mental framework within which the runes might be better appreciated. So far, so good. Then it seemed relevant to explore not only the mentality, but also the spirituality of that era, with the agency of the *soul* and to tease it out from our modern and Christian way of looking at both this and other spiritual concepts.

This had led us on a long journey away from the runes, but deeper into the mind and spirit of those who would have used them. I believe this is valid, because with this more authentic traditional – even ancestral – reconnection, the runes can be seen as quite integrated into the psycho-social milieu of the period. In this way, they parallel language, and with the absence of the written word, inform and be informed by and through oral tradition, narrative and mythology. When we get to explore magic in a bit more depth in the *Spellbinding* section, I trust this will all become more apparent.

However, before I do this, I would like to briefly look at a couple of themes related to the above apparent digressions, which also serve to link these discussions directly back to the Futhorc.

Runes, Tarot, Alchemy & the Holy Grail

This will be a somewhat speculative section; it conceptually arose during the writing of *Just Add Blood* and was one reason that I saw this earlier work to be relatively incomplete. There are some leaps of intuition – and faith – in what follows, so be warned! I also want to put this present study of the runes in context, as too often the subject is treated in isolation and connected to divination in a trivial manner; I want to redress some of this modern trend, as well as open up some lines of inquiry that may be of further interest.

It is no accident that I came to the runes by way of medicine and medical practice. I have a psychospiritual restlessness that meant I was always destined to explore the historical and archetypal undercurrents to medicine, health and healing, as well as my own personal place in this mix. In this process, I came across the runes through my own ancestral reconnection and exploration of my heritage. Initially this was in the context of Druidry in its traditional Celtic and reconstructionist context, but with an Anglo-Saxon continuation into the common and modern eras. And with this was a slightly more obscure connection – that there were Druids who could be identified as alchemists. In Welsh, they even had a name: *Pheryllt* or *Fferyllt*.

Alchemy is yet another tradition that existed before recorded history, from at least the advent of the metal Ages of Bronze and Iron. It is most commonly associated with what we refer to as the *Hermetic Tradition* and forms the basis of such arts and practices as medicine and magic (these two disciplines are not that dissimilar, by the way). Alchemy has an association with metals and the underground, and hence the vocational Blacksmith, often seen in a magical guise and in the figure of the Dwarf. It is also associated with astrology, as were the Druids, as well as the more esoteric medical traditions that have existed throughout time… from the shamanic archetype in prehistory, to such notable figures as the medieval Paracelsus, and the more modern figure of Jung.

For me, and for many years, the runes always had a slightly peripheral place. I was emotionally drawn to them and worked with them privately, but I did not see their relevance to my work as a medical practitioner – albeit with a holistic and psychotherapeutic orientation – until I left practice to pursue my psychospiritual interests more exclusively. It was then that things started to fall into place. Initially this was heralded by the rather enigmatic features I was gleaning in **Eolh** – ᛉ – and **Peorth** – ᛥ – not just with the interpretations, but also with their symbolic representation.

As I gravitated, or was 'pulled' toward the Old English Futhorc from the Germanic Elder Futhark – after a little detour through the Younger Futhark – I was particularly drawn to the latter runes of the Futhorc extension, the ones sometimes referred to as Northumbrian. Many threads that pulled me there, historical; my own heritage; the mystical exploration of the Grail; to mention but three. Yet I put all these on one side – relatively – until I had explored alchemy and its magical expression in greater depth. I had come home, because the symbolism of the Grail had held me in its thrall, permeated my dreams, and now emerged in the Philosopher's Stone. So, I returned to the runes.

This is, however, not a treatise on either alchemy, Hermeticism, magic, or medicine; it is about the runes. So, as I explore the relevant runes with extensions into these disciplines, and although they overlap, I will by necessity leave it to the reader to follow up the threads and connections that become relevant to them in their ongoing reading. Otherwise, I'll lose track and this work will become a monster of the non-mythological kind!

Prior to reading what follows, may I suggest looking back at both **Eolh** and **Peorth**, and at least taking on board the actual symbolic shapes of the two glyphs. In some ways, these glyphs weave their way through the Northumbrian extension, which is how I will refer to the last five or so runes, and ultimately into some sort of unity in **Gar**. As an example, look at them as a gender polarity, with **Eolh** as male and **Peorth** as female (or vice versa, if you prefer). Then look at the 'dance' that occurs through the Northumbrian extension. It could even be given a sexual connotation – alchemy would like that – with **Gar** being the outcome: The androgyne, Philosopher's Stone, or even the Holy Grail. But, I am getting ahead of myself…

Runes 28 – 31 (**Ior** to **Calc**) have elemental features: water, earth, fire and air (as spirit), if looked at successively and with a little latitude, as I have indicated here with **Calc**. I would also like to look at an alternative ordering with **Ior** and **Ear** exchanging places and hence the elemental order being earth > water > fire > air. I am doing this because it happens to align with the subtle progression of the elements, if looked at from a ritual and/or alchemical perspective. These are loose associations maybe, but they are interesting and quite suggestive of undercurrents that are not readily visible.

The basis of alchemy is a process. In very simple terms, the so-called *Work* is the transformation of the base metal, lead, into a noble one, gold. There is a physical aspect to this, but it is the more psychospiritual aspects that have risen to prominence, most notably with Jung and some of his followers. This sees the transformation as being the purification and perfection of man, in the true spiritual sense of that word.

The first phase of this, the *Lesser Work*, is where the elements clearly feature. The raw material (of the personality; maybe including Jung's concept of *shadow*) is contained, burnt, washed, the pure features identified and separated, then joined in a new and more evolved state of being characterised by the union of male and female in the individual personality. These stages are characterised by the elements, and these are clearly present in runes 28 – 31. **Calc** is notably an inverted **Eolh**, and is referred to as a cup, or chalice. The inversion may represent the embodiment of spirit within matter (the body).

The second phase is called the *Greater Work* and is more spiritual in orientation, in contrast to the more psychological Lesser Work. The stages are considered to be putrefaction/fermentation, distillation and then coagulation. I should point out that that these seven stages are generally acknowledged, although consistent with the relative obscurity of alchemy and its probably intentional obfuscation, there are all sorts of permutations and numbers of stages (maybe as many as there were alchemists).

A simplification of the seven-stage process outlined here, is a four stage one, roughly correlating to those of the Lesser Work, and colour-coded. Called nigredo > albedo > citrinas > rubedo after the Latin, the progression is black > white > yellow > red and encompasses the *Whole Work* that is both Lesser and Greater Works combined into one simplified proves. It is relatively easy to see an elemental association here, although the explanation of the colour red with air, or even fire as an alternative, would take us too far afield into the alchemical vaults for our current purposes.

If we are now dealing with the Greater Work in the Futhorc, there are only two runes left… or are there? I wonder whether the so-called **Double Calc** or **KK** – ᛤ – may actually herald the conjunction of male and female that characterises the completion of the Lesser Work, and that the inverted **Calc** – ᛣ – may symbolise the immersion into the stage of fermentation, sometimes recognised as putrefaction initially, rather like the physical process itself (as in brewing). If this is the case, then one part of the riddle of the latter runes might have a tentative solution.

Gar – ᚸ – is a spear, and the mystical association with the chalice is strong, both in Christianity (The Passion of Jesus Christ) and in the various Grail Legends, where they are incorporated into the ritual procession. I have put **Gar** here for a reason that we will come to shortly, but it is like a **Double Calc** without the central stave, maybe pure spirit minus the physical body? (Now I am being highly speculative.)

Stan – ᛥ – normally precedes **Gar**, but I have put the rune here at the end, because the *Philosopher's Stone* is the end point – the symbolic completion of the Work. There are a couple of other associations I would like to add, such as it is the stone from which the sword (Excalibur) is drawn in the Arthurian Legends. Also, **Stan** is like a 'completed' **Peorth**. Is **Peorth** the beginning of this process and hence misplaced in its common position? Does putting **Stan** at the end, indicate a deep feminine undercurrent to the process – as reflected in both the Arthurian and Grail Legends that has been usurped by putting **Gar** at the end?

How this applies to the Grail legends, I have hinted at but will not pursue in any detail here, as it forms a significant part of another work of mine, *The Charm of Making*. It is just that I firmly believe that the later runes of the Futhorc have alchemical significance, and that this theme is readily applicable to the Grail legends. In doing this, I am linking pre-Christian traditions with esoteric or mystical Christianity; something that has been done in other ways (mainly via the chalice), so my inquiry reinforces this. It also links mystical Christianity more firmly with Heathen

Tradition than its exoteric or religious structure does – but that's another story... as well as being an 'alchemical work in progress'!

The supposed *hallows* are commonly associated with Christianity, but in fact preceding it in Celtic and pre-Celtic traditions, such as with the quasi-historical and mythical *Tuatha De Denann* who supposedly brought these treasures to Ireland from Hyperborea, prior to the Celtic occupancy of that island. The hallows comprise the spear, sword, cup or chalice, dish or bowl and can be traced in the Futhorc, more significantly in the extension. However, these treasures also form the basis of the four suits of the Tarot known as the *Minor Arcana*, a word relatively synonymous with *rune* in meaning, as well as being the precursor modern playing cards. In the Minor Arcana there are fourteen cards per suit, being the addition of a *Page* to the court cards of King, Queen and Jack (or Knight) in the modern playing card pack. The Page may be the young apprentice to the Knight, but also – in alchemical fashion – his female consort.

Of further interest is that the Tarot also has twenty-two cards known as the *Major Arcana* that are commonly numbered, with the exception of the *Fool*, who is also rather anomalously present in the modern playing card pack as the *Joker*. The Major Arcana contains pictorial representations of what Jung would refer to as *archetypal images*. Combined with the Minor cards, whose meaning in the suits transcends numerical value, they could be seen as pathways of initiation and repositories of spiritual wisdom.

Although of a more recent historical period, the overlap with the Futharks, and most particularly the Futhorc and its extension, is significant and indicates these tools to be used in secret and mysterious ways throughout history, at the very least, and as an undercurrent to exoteric religious organisation, such as Christianity. They may even be the origin of the rather obscure books medieval writers and poets refer to as source material for their works to distance themselves from charges of magic from the Church establishment and its agency of the Inquisition.

There are these questions, and more. As stated, they are speculative and a product of my fertile imagination. But that is the nature of this work; it is about some sort of psychic archaeology as well as being to establish life and future into a traditional process. This section alone could be the subject of a separate work; it is necessarily a bit disjointed and incomplete. But it does indicate the level of inquiry that the runes can raise, as well as indicating they are not a separate feature of historical and idle curiosity, but a vital thread in a living Spiritual Tradition.

Spellbinding

This section will overlap earlier ones, particularly the section on *Magic* in the Religious and Spiritual Context (p127); please tolerate any duplication here and, as before, consider it as revision. It will also bring in topics previously referred to, such as charms, amulets, talismans etc., and put them in a more ritualised context. Naturally, this will extend to spells and the whole field of operative magic. It may also refer to contentious areas, such as drugs. Be warned.

How to approach this subject? It is better in-person and in workshops – that sort of setting. It wasn't because of any lack of capability that many traditions eschewed documented writing and relied on oral transmission; the word rune and its meanings implies it, after all. A lot can be lost or misinterpreted in translation, although I will accept the limitations of the exclusively written word and sketch an outline here. Of course, there are many ways to undertake this, even with the inherent type-written restrictions, but I want to approach the subject matter with a kind of modern feeling sensibility. Then, it may be possible to inquire into and explore the subject without the weight of evidence, information, academia and the like. What I also want the reader to do is to appreciate that we live in a cultural flatland; a kind of psychic two-dimensional reality. Everything from the past and the future is defined in terms of ourselves living in the material present. We lead a linear existence from birth to death, entrapped by the *machines* of our existence, be they material or immaterial.

If we were to explore magic in this manner within the present inquiry, I would probably have called this book *Spellbound* (please excuse any irony). But I have called it – and this section – *Spellbinding*; I am using other more flexible grammatical forms, instead of the exclusive fixity. I have taken the structured rigidity of the noun and liberated it, by applying fluidity and activity, as well as loosened up its boundaries. Elementally, I am using water rather than earth. Spellbound is fixed and can be entrapping; Spellbinding is empowering – can you feel the difference? We are defined and restricted by our physical existence, if we consider it only with nouns. Birth. Life. And death. So let us switch from fixed structure to dynamic process ...

Take *charm*. Now consider *charming*. If you consider a thing or a person to be charming, it or they have a certain quality, a feeling. This feeling is also associated with *power*. It or they are empowered and *empowering*, maybe toward or over you. The fact this is often considered in the realm of sexual dynamics is really no surprise. Experiment: Try and be charming ... use your voice and words, eyes and hands; see the effect on others. What about *enchantment?* This can also be disempowering, even spellbinding. The word *chant* refers to the voice, remember ... *Something* that is *enchanting* is powerful; it draws us toward it or them. But what about if we are enchanting, how does that feel? Objects, like *amulets* and *talismans* are an extension of this into craft, the hand. They also extend to the eyes, with sight. They may have a charm *chanted* into them, speech and voice. Play with these. Got the feeling and differences yet?

This is all the basis of *spells* and *spellcasting*. Don't forget that the process or activity mode of the fixity of spell is *spelling*. How close to the surface is all this depth, the third dimension below our flatland, our routine tick-tock existence? Quite close it seems. Spelling is power, it *names* something. Naming is considered power. We name our animals, but also our cars, our houses ... our children. So, a spell is something heard or written, voiced or crafted. But it is something that involves and invokes power, and where this power resides and with what intent; these forces determine the spell. Are you getting a feel for this yet? Do you see – feel – why I am expressing these things this way, not as definitions and in categories?

I mentioned earlier that it was human functions like sight, speech, and the use of the hand that distinguishes us from other animals. To these, and inferred by speech, hearing should be added. Now all of these are present in this arena that is Spellbinding. Added to this are various mental functions, like vision extended to imagination, and hearing to music, creativity etc. Whilst I have focused on some of the limitations earlier in our mental make-up, these are often complemented by these other more creative, artistic, and intuitive abilities; the so-called higher mental functions, if we are of an Anglo-Saxon or similar disposition.

Now it can be seen that writing – or carving, engraving etc. – is an extension of these mental functions, and can include the higher creative and artistic ones. Are these present in the Roman script, or in Modern English? Vaguely sometimes (most of us learnt the alphabet with pictures …), but they have largely fallen or been stripped away; their complexity and dimensionality has been reduced. Obviously, this whole process is lengthy and complex, but let me give a few pointers.

I believe that the Roman civilisation – if you can call it civilised – has a lot to answer for, particularly when compared to the preceding and neighbouring Greek one. The Romans effectively decimated the existing Celtic culture in much of Britain, and this was then followed up by the adoption and extension of Roman power with its Church. In various forms, I argue that this more subtle political and social dominating force is still present, and disrupting our connection to our innate ancestral and spiritual heritage. The Roman script has served to continue and perpetuate this process, stripping the written word of depth and the other associated functions, outlined immediately above.

There is a subtle point that needs reinforcing here; that is, we have retained Old English as the spoken word into modernity; it has spread across the globe. Yet whilst we did not change to Latin as a language, we did adopt the Roman script. This is a further reason that oral transmission is more powerful and retained by spiritual and other esoteric practitioners, in prayer, ritual etc. The written word can lack the depth and complexity from other attributes, such as bodily expression, change in pitch, tone and cadence etc., which can accompany verbal utterance that the written word cannot. Instead, the written word in Modern English relies on analogy, euphemism, metaphor and symbol to achieve this; it requires a poetic disposition, in my opinion ... and Woden was that.

The runes retain many of these functions and have, in fact, accompanied them in our human evolution; they are its mirror and expression. Their roots are in the metaphysical realms of our existence and our manifestation into physical form. They are the *words* of the gods, whatever the latter might be. Unlike Roman letters that have been stripped of it, they express power and intent. Of course, the runes can be used for the same purposes that we use modern language for now – information, legal, institutional – but to confine them as this, as some commentators mistakenly do, is to simply see them as a competitor to the Roman script.

I do not hold to that view, either in my research or personal experience; runes are representative of this more three-dimensional reality that includes depth, and much more beyond. And it is this *more* that I am attempting to convey here, which I believe has been repressed by the dominant and controlling influences in our modern two thousand year's history. Nothing else as well explains the mess modernity is in. It is no wonder to me that the runes have resurfaced and are being used by people like me: And I hardly consider myself a New Age devotee.

But I don't need to convince you. As meditation teachers tell us, the evidence that meditation *works* is in the practice, and not the theory or the science, which are merely explanations of the fact that it does work. Consider the runes in a similar way; try using them to see if they work. That is why I wrote the *how to ...* section, even though – in a written work like this – it has its limitations; as, indeed, does this section. It comes down to practice and experimentation. You need to walk your talk, because the map is not the territory.

How to use runes for spells? Start off with a question maybe, and do a reading. See the outcome in the way I have already described. Does it answer your question? This route is fairly simple, unambiguous, and does not directly involve power or necessarily another person. A bit like praying, really. The dialogue between you and the unknown is also fairly clear; you are a bit more involved in the process than praying, and the means that you use – the runes – provide a particular seemingly limited range of responses. However, the psychic extension of these approaches and their responses is itself unlimited.

How about something different. You are looking for a particular outcome in the world, like a love-match or a career change, and want to influence the process. Now things are getting a bit deeper. What is your intent, and are your motives pure and free or personal investment, like control or manipulation? Be aware that the outcome may be as you *desired* but not necessarily in the way you wanted. As an example, I once had a vintage car I really liked and cast a spell that I would never receive a speeding ticket when I drove it. I never did; instead, the car was written off in a road accident some years later.

If your knowledge of the runes is good, you may want to construct something with them to use as a kind of spell. Now you are more involved with the process, so self-responsibility increases. Factors like direction and purpose, desire and need, determination and power all enter the equation. In my opinion, we need to closely examine our individual motive for a spell and why we are using it, beyond more mundane methods of effecting an outcome. If not, the darker side of spellcasting comes into play, and this has a very enigmatic history. Read *Faust*.

Runes can exist in combinations, bound, in a similar way to letters forming words, except more holistic and powerful. If you look at your rune set now, you can easily see that some runes resemble and even contain others, such as **Lagu** in **Eoh**, or both **Eh** and **Wyn** in **Man**. I have drawn on the significance of some of this in the discussion of individual runes. But here we are talking about something different; how to combine runes into a new and (relatively) unique form, knowing that there are various outcomes and these could in themselves be significant; particularly as the combination often contains runes that were not initially part of the process, which may carry a further and differing significance.

This process is making *bindrunes*, the binding together of individual runes, that in itself can be the result of divining and casting a spell; please be aware of the difference between divining and *casting*, the latter is what we can do with a bindrune. This can be creating a charm, engraving a stone or other object, sacrificing anything created to fire, wind and water … the combinations are endless and in your hands. I described one such bindrune earlier in the book, but did not draw it pictorially. I will not be doing that here, as I would be committing a spell process to paper, this book. And, given that the end of a spell is often the sacrifice of the bindrune (to fire or water), then it would be inappropriate. It is also up to you to practice.

I am aware that these remarks are necessarily limited, although deliberately and inevitably so. As a practising medicine man, or shaman, I am mindful of the ethics I operate within. I believe there is more than enough said already to start the interested participant off on a magical path, or at least to use the runes more magically and spiritually within their own practice. This is the point that instruction almost demands a teacher or mentor, although this is not a prerequisite. I have not had one for the runes and operative magical practice, although I have had extensive training in several disciplines that support this work. I act on my own authority.

Is this hubris? Many, many years ago I was told that a journalist had met with some aboriginal elders in a Kimberley community, which had a strong magical tradition, and asked them why they were not teaching their young people. The response was something like, "because new laws coming". I suspect they *saw* in the visionary sense that which we are now experiencing. Our Eldership initiation is from the process itself, and the figures we encounter there; we are learning and developing traditional patterns with a kind of retrieval and reconstruction process, and not shirking the demand because we are decimated of immediate physical eldership. We are learning from each other, our responsibility is to teach, as well as to serve our community.

I am conscious of power. In our society, we too readily cede power to those who demand it for their own self-aggrandisement, as well as for the manipulation and control of others, based on our own fears and needs. We need to acknowledge power in ourselves for our own purpose and direction, because a life without it is one unlived, in my opinion. And denying it means we either transfer it to others (often inappropriately) or repress it in ourselves, when it can then operate in sometimes disturbing ways, such as self-sabotage, trauma, or in disease manifestation.

Maybe bindrunes need a little more explanation; bearing in mind that this section is entirely my own, with its deductions and interpretations. Hopefully, you will have become a bit more familiar by now with using runes in combination, as with any divinatory readings, and started to experiment with bindrunes, particularly if your interest is spells and magic. If not, and anyway, you may want to play with combinations and bindrunes by laying out a set, putting various combinations together, and then maybe drawing a bindrune or bindrunes (there are usually several potential combinations). Then explore what the bindrune may have captured, in terms of other runes not originally used in the initial combination. This may be of hidden or deeper import and is always worth paying attention to.

Drawing a parallel with Modern English, there is a kind of syntax. However, always – always – remember that the runes are not simple letters, particularly of the Roman script, they carry a metaphoric and symbolic depth relatively denied in the latter. But maybe as a metaphor this syntax interpretation stands, where the runes are letters or combinations of letters, and the readings are phrases or sentences. They are like a statement rather than a story; it is our responsibility to weave them into a narrative for our lives.

Then a bindrune could be considered like a dream, or a condensation of the story created. It is a result of the dialogue between you and the unknown, an expression of the *Ground of Being*. Even consider it like an artwork, a painting; but remember, these are metaphors. Yet they are useful, as they take us out of our linear time-ordered way of thinking about the runes, divinatory readings, and magical acts. They become a language or, more truly, a metalanguage that is the expression of the narrative of life.

Then bindrunes can be seen as magical, and used in practice. Taking them into ritual honours and expresses them, it gives them power. Then applying our *intent* in the form of a spell or charm gives the bindrune wings for expression and – the gods willing – to align with your will and intended outcome. Although always remember, it may be thus, but not the way you might previously have thought or in the manner you wanted! Magic is an art, and it is by our mistakes we learn. But this is where practice is important, and personal guidance, if available and preferably in-person; your own counsel may be a better guide than the internet!

Take a breath …

Having arrived at this point and written this book, I have already asked what comes next, and have two answers (at least). The first is a more practical work, called *Sacred Space*, which I am using as the basis of ritual and ceremonial work in my individual work and the community network I operate within. This extends through ritual to an Anglo-Celtic rendering of the Sweat House ceremonial process. Whilst presently restricted to oral teaching and its online extension, as well as my counselling work, it is gradually developing into a book. And the runes are an integral part of this and, at the very least, *Sacred Space* will become a complementary work to this one.

As my work develops, an increasing amount of it is conducted in a ritual and sometimes ceremonial context. In fact, it is only the more peripheral health counselling work that stands outside, although even with this I like to engage in a mutually conducive setting. So, if not formally ritualised, it is usually in a natural setting or location. This is because I consider the setting an important part of healing work, even if only counselling; if more therapeutic, then I use a more formal ritual structure.

Healing is an integral part of rune work, as is ritual. So, it makes sense that if healing is the focus of any encounter, then not only a ritual setting, but also a ritual format is often employed. This is certainly the case if runes are used in the therapeutic encounter. When considered in this broader manner, it is evident that ritual is a relatively lost art in modernity, replaced by blind regimentation and confining ritual process to the underworld or the nursery, where it can emerge in patterns of psychological distress. Often not considered appropriately, such unawares ritual process contains the content demanding to be brought to light and healed.

This is so often the case when health concerns indicate a disease process. In the anxiety that any severe disease produces – particularly if death is a possible consequence – the mental framework of the sufferer often becomes quite naturally ritualised. If the content of this could be explored in either a direct or symbolic manner, then alternative and more healing approaches could be utilised. In fact, the loss of ritual process is broader and includes our modern culture, such that the disease process itself may be drawing us into healing not only the disease, but the broader psycho-social context in which it emerged.

Runes are an integral part of the healing process, when applicable. This may be simply for divinatory purposes, but can extend to a more visionary and prophetic role. Spell-making and casting, often employing bindrunes, is a powerful adjunct. But this is not conducted in isolation, it is an integral part of the ritual process of healing and intimately connected with the client's narrative. Ultimately, this process must be conducted in such a way that the power balance is equitable and the flow creative and purposeful, from which direction will flow.

I would make some brief comment on sex and drugs. I have made some reference to sexuality at various points, particularly where I see it to be embedded in the runes themselves; which I believe it is. Yet, more than this, I see a specific role for the use of sexuality with the runes, as well as within magical practice more generally. With a discerning eye, sexual patterns can be seen in individual runes. It is then a natural and magical extension to see and experiment with them in ritual combination, even as bindrunes.

Sexuality is an extremely powerful tool and really cannot be ignored in any study of such topics as spirituality, magic, and associated disciplines like alchemy. My position currently is to view sexuality and spirituality as synonymous; two sides of the same coin. I would further mention that traditional societies are more able to differentiate the social, family, and spiritual roles of sexuality better than most in the modern West. This extends to an appreciation of different patterns of sexual relations that includes orgiastic behaviour. This topic is a book in itself; I mention it not only for completion, but to encourage its active engagement by you, the reader, if not already done so.

With drugs, I am talking mainly of the natural and hallucinogenic variety, *medicine*, if you will. Herein, I also include alcohol and nicotine; both are used in many cultures in ceremony. The tobacco plant can be used as a medicine. Similarly, we have lost the creative and therapeutic art associated with alcohol, not to mention its connection with other drugs for which it can be used as a carrier medium. Certainly, the social and ritual use of alcohol has become progressively less appreciated in the modern era.

Hallucinogenic drugs are a powerful adjunct to ritual and the facilitation of visionary, prophetic and healing experiences through altered states of consciousness. These drugs are an integral part of the shaman's medicine bag and are often used in ceremony, as with ayahuasca. Hallucinogenic mushrooms are used worldwide. These are sparse comments that serve to highlight the significance of drugs, but also my endorsement of their use in appropriate settings under ritual conditions, other restrictions notwithstanding.

Such matters should be in the hands of initiated elders and healers – effectively the shamans – and not the political, legal and even medical authorities of our time. They are powerful and not playthings, but will be used indiscriminately as such if suppressed, leading to unpredictable health consequences and social problems. They are probably the most effective tool in the treatment of mental health in the West that is being actively ignored, or being given to inappropriate agencies like the Pharmaceutical Industry and the medical profession, rather than true healers.

Sex and drugs lead us, directly or indirectly, into the *altered state of consciousness* world of the shaman. An exploration of the runes, undertaken in ritual circumstances, can lead to a similar result. What will support and facilitate this process is the creative and active use of the imagination. Vision, prophesy and seership are abilities latent within us all. They require training and practice to develop, but the imagination is an indispensable tool in this process (and dreamwork is a good place to start). Not only is imagination the language that we use for these tools, it is also the way the transpersonal, archetypal reality – the *gods* if you like – communicate to us.

Interestingly to me is that hallucinogens not only gain access to altered states of consciousness with its visionary expression, but also to the mental patterns that appear to underlie conscious experience. Specifically, with some such as DMT – a component both of ayahuasca and also a constituent of the pineal gland in the brain – are geometric shapes. It is not a far step to see this stratum of consciousness as the foundation of the runes themselves, such that the individual runes are truly a gift of the gods and not simply a product of trivial human imagination or the desire to communicate in a scriptural manner.

So, where is my practical and ritual life going in my research and writing as I come to the completion of this book? I am working on practical bindrune extensions beyond magical usage, as well as creating my own rune row. Using the 33-34 Futhorc rune row as a base, I am using the bindrune principle to condense the runes into a more dense and symbolic form for more extended magical purposes, such as in the naming of people and locations.

Further, and similar to the way the Younger developed from the Elder Futhark, I am working my own reduced rune row set, maybe 16 or so; although the runes themselves may have something to say in this. It is also something I will experiment with and use practically, before writing about the process and result. This is currently a work in progress, and I hope to accompany it poetically by writing my own rune poems, with a little *galdic* inspiration, of course!

I have utilised the word *spellbinding* here in both its literal and metaphoric sense. Although somewhat restricted by the medium of words written in a book, I have tried to include within this restraint what has been necessarily omitted; being voice, hearing, and further creative expression. However, I trust that enough has been inferred to engage the reader's imagination and desire to explore this territory further.

Maybe the way to appreciate *spellbinding* in this expanded manner is through the metaphoric and symbolic expression of the word, as well as the way it is engaged. To do this, it may help to recall the varying facets of the Anglo-Saxon Mentality and look almost *around* the word itself. Feel it … it is magical. It draws in the imagination, and stimulates creativity. Intuitively, it draws you back into past eras with its mythic and folkloric attraction. In contrast, spiritually it is challenging by engaging the apparent darkness of magic in the word itself, with its erotic and almost sadomasochistic overtones. But in so doing, it invites its opposite, with play in the lightness of being. By poetic expression, in opposition and contrast, it is, in itself, magic.

Postscript

Ultimately, if runes are taken out of the exclusively academic and research arenas, they can only be fully appreciated in the context of magic; which is what I have attempted to do here. It is not that I reject these other disciplines and their associated sciences, it is just that we have taken this part of the entire picture and made it the whole by excluding other positions and their input. In effect, I have called this reductive position flatland, and given it a metaphoric two-dimensional visual picture, where the third dimension of depth has been excluded; not to mention the dimensions beyond that approach the ground of being, and which can be collectively referred to as spiritual.

In my work, I use the following prayer in ritual and ceremony:

> May the ground of all being,
> Guide me/us in thought, word and deed,
> Now and forevermore.
>
> A'rún

I want to focus on the "thought, word and deed," and its relevance: I feel the "ground of all being," aspect has been covered. Equivalent to the Christian *amen*, or the Celtic druidic *awen*, "A'rún" is our equivalent, where *rún* refers to the rune of secrecy or whisper.

Thought as idea, word in speech or written, is the basis of deed or action; or as I have mentioned, it is "walking our talk". From a magical perspective thoughts and words are dynamic and can be used to engage the metaphysical reality – in whatever way we envision it – in a dialogue, as the basis of magic. We can do this in a spell, or a charm, as well as other spoken, chanted or creative acts, such the making of a talisman or amulet. This is an act of faith based on more than belief, but in a Gnostic kind of *knowing*.

In *Spellbinding*, I have explored the nature of the runes from the original work as a kind of *how to* ... and extended that to bring in related fields in the psychospiritual domains to support my thesis. But ultimately magic depends on you, and how you use it. The runes are one way that I find significant because of my ancestry and heritage, but there are others; there is no exclusive path to the top of the mountain, although the mountain top is common.

Travel well.

Appendices

A glance at the first appendix partially amends my rather restricted reference to date regarding the phonetic aspects of the runes, although the reason for this relative omission was discussed and explained earlier. In this appendix I have added the phonetic value of the 33 runes of the Futhorc to the graphic symbol and its name, then followed this with a similar description of both the Elder and Younger Futharks.

This addition may be useful if you have only an Elder Futhark rune row to work with, or if you choose this as a viable option. But the appendix is also designed to give an outline of the three rune rows of the Futharks for comparative purposes, as these form the basis of our modern appreciation of the runic corpus.

Please do not be under the modern tendency and belief that this or any study will provide a unified picture. You may have appreciated by now that there is a considerable variation in the Futhorc and this only increases when the remaining two other Futharks are considered. Instead, we have a rich and varied field, with many branches and strands. Our modern appreciation in general, and mine in particular, is simply an ongoing part of this fluid and creative process.

Instead, it can be seen that each feature – symbol, name, and phonetic value (plus the meanings outlined above and in the poems) – can be explored in its own right. The symbols and names have an overall cohesion, particularly when considered over time, although some retain a consistency whilst others become much more varied.

The phonetic values connect the runes with their use as an alphabet, yet also expands this to their common usage as a script and for communication, whereas the symbols and names take on a more esoteric and magical usage.

There is still a lot of disagreement regarding phonetics, and I have had to bite the bullet and chose one approach in the tables below; this is a system you may wish to modify from personal research and experience, and this is entirely valid: I contend this is a living Tradition. This philological approach is also of great value in the extended exploration of the runes beyond their magical usage.

An interesting and intriguing exercise is to explore this network of inter-relationships between the differing rune rows of the Futharks, as well as over the time period of their evolution. For example, the phonetic values give some indication of how the Elder was reduced in number to the Younger Futhark, and where omitted runes gained different associations in those retained. Additionally, runes can be given differing phonetic values, particularly when the vowels are considered.

This exercise can be extended to the symbols and names, because I have taken only one theme in several possible ones here, as well as with the phonetic values. For example, many rune shapes have alternatives. In the Futhorc the **Ing** rune may lack extensions upward and downwards to the left and right. Both **Ur** and **Sigel** can be shaped slightly differently. The changes to **Ing** and **Ur** are reflected in the alternative font I have used for the runes in the tables that follow, **Sigel** can be rotated a little clockwise to look like an angular modern 'S'. Similarly with the names, **Wyn** can be **Wynn**, **Sigel** can be **Sigil**, and **Hagal** can be **Haegl** as discussed. So, as well as the philological approach, an etymological study can be undertaken.

To explore all this, you may need lots of paper and coloured pens, as well as access to the reference books in the index;

because I have taken a fairly single and somewhat arbitrary line through these various options according to personal inclination.

As hinted at with the phonetic values, there are wider connections that can be considered. In the Futhorc, this becomes more obvious with the Northumbrian rune extension, where cultural and religious issues start to become more obvious. Also, some symbols get more focus and attention, as well as some starting to look more like bindrunes than single runes.

Ultimately the runes must be considered in this wider cultural context, as well as with the cultures that preceded their clear manifestation and continued in parallel with their influence. Remembering, of course, that our culture is having an active influence on the appreciation of the runes and their further development into the future.

Runelore remains a work in progress.

Anglo-Saxon Futhorc

NAME	PHONETIC VALUE	RUNE
Feoh	f	ᚠ
Ur	u	ᚢ
Thorn	th	ᚦ
Os	o	ᚩ
Rad	r	ᚱ
Cen	c (k)	ᚳ
Gyfu	g	ᚷ
Wyn	w	ᚹ
Hagal	h	ᚻ
Nyd	n	ᚾ
Is	i	ᛁ
Ger	y	ᛄ
Eoh	eo	ᛇ
Peorth	p	ᛈ
Eolh	x/z	ᛉ
Sigel	s	ᛋ

Tir	t	↑
Beorc	b	ᛒ
Eh	e	ᛖ
Man	m	ᛗ
Lagu	l	ᛚ
Ing	ng	◇
Ethel	e (oe)	ᛟ
Daeg	d	ᛞ
Ac	a	ᚪ
Aesc	ae	ᚫ
Yr	y	ᛦ
Ior	eo (io)	⁎
Ear	ea	ᛠ
Cweorth	q	ᛢ
Calc	k	ᛣ alt ᛤ
Stan	st	ᛥ
Gar	(g)	ᚸ

Elder Futhark

NAME	PHONETIC VALUE	RUNE
Fehu	f	ᚠ
Uruz	u	ᚢ
Thurisaz	th	ᚦ
Ansuz	a	ᚨ
Raido	r	ᚱ
Kenaz	k	ᚲ
Gebo	g	ᚷ
Wunjo	w	ᚹ
Hagalaz	h	ᚺ
Nauthiz	n	ᚾ
Isa	i	ᛁ
Jera	j	ᛃ
Eiwaz	i/e	ᛇ
Pertho	p	ᛈ
Algiz	z/r	ᛉ
Sowilo	s	ᛋ

Tiwaz	t	↑
Berkano	b	ᛒ
Ehwaz	e	ᛖ
Mannaz	m	ᛗ
Laguz	l	ᛚ
Ingwaz	ng	◇
Othala	o	ᛟ
Dagaz	d	ᛞ

Younger Futhark

NAME	PHONETIC VALUE	RUNE
Fe	f	ᚠ
Ur	u/o/v	ᚢ
Thurs	th/dh	ᚦ
Ass	a	ᚨ
Reidh	r	ᚱ
Kaun	k/g/ng	ᚴ
Hagall	h	ᚼ
Naudh	n	ᚾ
Iss	i/e	ᛁ
Ar	a	ᛅ
Sol	s	ᛋ
Tyr	t/d/nd	ᛏ
Bjarkan	b/p	ᛒ
Madhr	m	ᛘ
Logr	l	ᛚ
Yr	-R	ᛦ

The Anglo-Saxon Rune Poem

Feoh
Wealth is a comfort to all men;
yet must every man bestow it freely,
if he wish to gain honour in the sight of the Lord.

Ur
The aurochs is proud and has great horns;
it is a very savage beast and fights with its horns;
a great ranger of the moors, it is a creature of mettle.

Thorn
The thorn is exceedingly sharp,
an evil thing for any knight to touch,
uncommonly severe on all who sit among them.

Os
The mouth is the source of all language,
a pillar of wisdom and a comfort to wise men,
a blessing and a joy to every knight.

Rad
Riding seems easy to every warrior while he is indoors
and very courageous to him who traverses the high-roads
on the back of a stout horse.

Cen
The torch is known to every living man by its pale, bright flame;
it always burns where princes sit within.

Gyfu
Generosity brings credit and honour, which support one's dignity;
it furnishes help and subsistence
to all broken men who are devoid of aught else.

Wynn
Bliss he enjoys who knows not suffering, sorrow nor anxiety,
and has prosperity and happiness and a good enough house.

Haegl
Hail is the whitest of grain;
it is whirled from the vault of heaven
and is tossed about by gusts of wind
and then it melts into water.

Nyd
Trouble is oppressive to the heart;
yet often it proves a source of help and salvation
to the children of men, to everyone who heeds it betimes.

Is
Ice is very cold and immeasurably slippery;
it glistens as clear as glass and most like to gems;
it is a floor wrought by the frost, fair to look upon.

Ger
Summer is a joy to men, when God, the holy King of Heaven,
suffers the earth to bring forth shining fruits
for rich and poor alike.

Eoh
The yew is a tree with rough bark,
hard and fast in the earth, supported by its roots,
a guardian of flame and a joy upon an estate.

Peordh
Peorth is a source of recreation and amusement to the great,
where warriors sit blithely together in the banqueting-hall.

Eolh
The Eolh-sedge is mostly to be found in a marsh;
it grows in the water and makes a ghastly wound,
covering with blood every warrior who touches it.

Sigel
The sun is ever a joy in the hopes of seafarers
when they journey away over the fishes' bath,
until the courser of the deep bears them to land.

Tir
Tiw is a guiding star; well does it keep faith with princes;
it is ever on its course over the mists of night and never fails.

Beorc
The poplar bears no fruit; yet without seed it brings forth suckers,
for it is generated from its leaves.
Splendid are its branches and gloriously adorned
its lofty crown which reaches to the skies.

Eh
The horse is a joy to princes in the presence of warriors.
A steed in the pride of its hoofs,
when rich men on horseback bandy words about it;
and it is ever a source of comfort to the restless.

Mann
The joyous man is dear to his kinsmen;
yet every man is doomed to fail his fellow,
since the Lord by his decree will commit the vile carrion to the earth.

Lagu
The ocean seems interminable to men,
if they venture on the rolling bark
and the waves of the sea terrify them
and the courser of the deep heed not its bridle.

Ing
Ing was first seen by men among the East-Danes,
till, followed by his chariot,
he departed eastwards over the waves.
So the Heardingas named the hero.

Ethel
An estate is very dear to every man,
if he can enjoy there in his house
whatever is right and proper in constant prosperity.

Dæg
Day, the glorious light of the Creator, is sent by the Lord;
it is beloved of men, a source of hope and happiness to rich and poor,
and of service to all.

Ac
The oak fattens the flesh of pigs for the children of men.
Often it traverses the gannet's bath,
and the ocean proves whether the oak keeps faith
in honourable fashion.

Æsc
The ash is exceedingly high and precious to men.
With its sturdy trunk it offers a stubborn resistance,
though attacked by many a man.

Yr

Yr is a source of joy and honour to every prince and knight;
it looks well on a horse and is a reliable equipment for a journey.

Ior

Iar is a river fish and yet it always feeds on land;
it has a fair abode encompassed by water, where it lives in happiness.

Ear

The grave is horrible to every knight,
when the corpse quickly begins to cool
and is laid in the bosom of the dark earth.
Prosperity declines, happiness passes away
and covenants are broken.

The Norse Rune Poem

Fe
Wealth is a source of discord among kinsmen;
the wolf lives in the forest.

Ur
Dross comes from bad iron;
the reindeer often races over the frozen snow.

Thurs
Giant causes anguish to women;
misfortune makes few men cheerful.

As
Estuary is the way of most journeys;
but a scabbard is of swords.

Reidh
Riding is said to be the worst thing for horses;
Reginn forged the finest sword.

Kaun
Ulcer is fatal to children;
death makes a corpse pale.

Hagall
Hail is the coldest of grain;
Christ created the world of old.

Naudhr
Constraint gives scant choice;
a naked man is chilled by the frost.

Isa
Ice we call the broad bridge;
the blind man must be led.

Ar
Plenty is a boon to men;
I say that Frodi was generous.

Sol
Sun is the light of the world;
I bow to the divine decree.

Tyr
Tyr is a one-handed god;
often has the smith to blow.

Bjarkan
Birch has the greenest leaves of any shrub;
Loki was fortunate in his deceit.

Madhr
Man is an augmentation of the dust;
great is the claw of the hawk.

Logr
A waterfall is a River which falls from a mountain-side;
but ornaments are of gold.

Yr
Yew is the greenest of trees in winter;
it is wont to crackle when it burns.

The Icelandic Rune Poem

Fé – Wealth
Source of discord among kinsmen
and fire of the sea
and path of the serpent.

Úr – Shower
Lamentation of the clouds
and ruin of the hay-harvest
and abomination of the shepherd.

Thurs – Giant
Torture of women
and cliff-dweller
and husband of a giantess.

Óss – God
Aged Gautr
and prince of Ásgardr
and lord of Vallhalla.

Reid – Riding
Joy of the horsemen
and speedy journey
and toil of the steed.

Kaun – Ulcer
Disease fatal to children
and painful spot
and abode of mortification.

Hagall – Hail
Cold grain
and shower of sleet
and sickness of serpents.

Naud – Constraint
Grief of the bond-maid
and state of oppression
and toilsome work.

Iss – Ice
Bark of rivers
and roof of the wave
and destruction of the doomed.

Ár – Plenty
Boon to men
and good summer
and thriving crops.

Sól – Sun
Shield of the clouds
and shining ray
and destroyer of ice.

Tyr
God with one hand
and leavings of the wolf
and prince of temples.

Bjarken – Birch
Leafy twig
and little tree

and fresh young shrub.

Maðr – Man
Delight of man
and augmentation of the earth
and adorner of ships.

Lögr – Water
Eddying stream
and broad geyser
and land of the fish.

Yr – Yew
Bent bow
and brittle iron
and giant of the arrow.

(From "Runic and Heroic Poems" by Bruce Dickins)

Havamal

Odin

Wounded I hung on a wind-swept gallows
For nine long nights,
Pierced by a spear, pledged to Odhinn,
Offered, myself to myself
The wisest know not from whence spring
The roots of that ancient rood
They gave me no bread,
They gave me no mead,
I looked down;
with a loud cry
I took up runes;
from that tree I fell.
Nine lays of power
I learned from the famous Bolthor, Bestla's father:
He poured me a draught of precious mead,
Mixed with magic Odrerir.
Waxed and throve well;
Word from word gave words to me,
Deed from deed gave deeds to me,
Runes you will find, and readable staves,
Very strong staves,
Very stout staves,
Staves that Bolthor stained,
Made by mighty powers,
Graven by the prophetic god,
For the gods by Odhinn, for the elves by Dain,

By Dvalin, too, for the dwarves,
By Asvid for the hateful giants,
And some I carved myself:
Thund, before man was made, scratched them,
Who rose first, fell thereafter
Know how to cut them, know how to read them,
Know how to stain them, know how to prove them,
Know how to evoke them, know how to score them,
Know how to send them "know how to send them,
Better not to ask than to over-pledge
As a gift that demands a gift"
Better not to send than to slay too many,
The first charm I know is unknown to rulers
Or any of human kind;
Help it is named,
for help it can give in hours of sorrow and anguish.
I know a second that the sons of men
Must learn who wish to be leeches.
I know a third: in the thick of battle,
If my need be great enough,
It will blunt the edges of enemy swords,
Their weapons will make no wounds.
I know a fourth:
it will free me quickly
If foes should bind me fast
With strong chains, a chant that makes Fetters spring from the feet,
Bonds burst from the hands.
I know a fifth: no flying arrow,
Aimed to bring harm to men,
Flies too fast for my fingers to catch it
And hold it in mid-air.
I know a sixth:
it will save me if a man

Cut runes on a sapling's Roots
With intent to harm; it turns the spell;
The hater is harmed, not me.
If I see the hall
Ablaze around my bench mates,
Though hot the flames, they shall feel nothing,
If I choose to chant the spell.
I know an eighth:
that all are glad of,
Most useful to men:
If hate fester in the heart of a warrior,
It will soon calm and cure him.
I know a ninth:
when need I have
To shelter my ship on the flood,
The wind it calms, the waves it smoothes
And puts the sea to sleep,
I know a tenth:
if troublesome ghosts
Ride the rafters aloft,
I can work it so they wander astray,
Unable to find their forms,
Unable to find their homes.
I know an eleventh:
when I lead to battle old comrades in-arms,
I have only to chant it behind my shield,
And unwounded they go to war,
Unwounded they come from war,
U unscathed wherever they are.
I know a twelfth:
If a tree bear
A man hanged in a halter,
I can carve and stain strong runes
That will cause the corpse to speak,

Reply to whatever I ask.
I know a thirteenth
if I throw a cup Of water over a warrior,
He shall not fall in the fiercest battle,
Nor sink beneath the sword,
I know a fourteenth, that few know:
If I tell a troop of warriors
About the high ones, elves and gods,
I can name them one by one.
(Few can the nit-wit name.)
I know a fifteenth,
that first Thjodrerir
Sang before Delling's doors,
Giving power to gods, prowess to elves,
Fore-sight to Hroptatyr Odhinn,
I know a sixteenth:
if I see a girl
With whom it would please me to play,
I can turn her thoughts, can touch the heart
Of any white armed woman.
I know a seventeenth:
if I sing it,
the young Girl will be slow to forsake me.
I know an eighteenth that I never tell
To maiden or wife of man,
A secret I hide from all
Except the love who lies in my arms,
Or else my own sister.
To learn to sing them, Loddfafnir,
Will take you a long time,
Though helpful they are if you understand them,
Useful if you use them,
Needful if you need them.
The Wise One has spoken words in the hall,

Needful for men to know,
Unneedful for trolls to know:
Hail to the speaker,
Hail to the knower,
Joy to him who has understood,
Delight to those who have listened.

(W. H. Auden & P. B. Taylor Translation)

Bibliography

General Runelore

Aswynn, Freya. *Northern Mysteries & Magick*. St. Paul, Llewellyn Publications, 2002
Fries, Jan. *Helrunar: A Handbook of Rune Magick*. Oxford, Mandrake, 2006
Thorsson, Edred. *Runelore*. York Beach, Samuel Weiser Inc. 1987
Thorsson, Edred. *Futhark: A Handbook of Rune Magic*. York Beach, Samuel Weiser Inc. 1984

Anglo-Saxon Runes

Albertsson, Alaric. *Wyrdworking: The Path of a Saxon Sorcerer*. Woodbury, Llewellyn, 2011
Bates, Brian. *The Way of Wyrd*. Carlsbad, Hay House, 2005
Elliott, RWV. *Runes: An Introduction*. Westport, Greenwood Press, 1959
Page, RI. *An Introduction to English Runes*. Woodbridge, Boydell Press, 2006
Pennick, Nigel. *Rune Magic: The History and Practice of Ancient Runic Traditions*. London, Thorsons, 1995
Tyson, Donald. *Rune Magic*. St. Paul, Llewellyn, 1995

This is but a brief outline of the runic corpus.

All books are about runes, with some extension. The exception is Brian Bates' *Way of Wyrd*, which has been included because it is a vivid portrayal of the Anglo-Saxon world and has a large bibliography.

The general books are based on the Elder Futhark and give a sound introduction with many avenues of exploration. The Futhorc Anglo-Saxon works are solely academic (Page), or with a contrasting and significantly broader appreciation and insight (Elliott), extending to the more familiar, yet differing styles of Pennick, Albertsson, and Tyson.

These writers were also chosen as they are significant in the field, and can be used to source further material in the disciplines that suit the reader. There are many possible avenues to explore from here, but this material will provide the road maps.

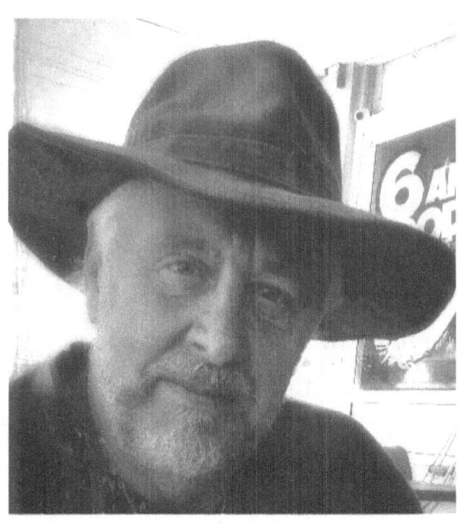

Biography

My work is with the recovery and reinstatement of the soul, individually and within our modern culture.

By my degrees, qualification and experience, I am an Oxford and London trained physiologist and medical doctor; by training and former practice a Jungian analyst; by initiation a Druid and shamanic healer; by decree an ordained priest and an elder in my tradition, and by disposition an alchemist, poet and wordsmith.

My former work as a general practitioner, holistic physician, and medical psychotherapist has been a preparation for this present path.

I am called to wrest from obscurity the ground between a dying religion, and a soul-less science ….

Volumes of knowledge and experience to be shared and dispensed to those who ask, and would listen.

An alchemist's robe I wrap around an ageing frame, a magical staff to feel my way, my heart beating to an ancient tune. A poetic sensibility is my torch.

A call to healing, vision and re-enchantment, a social cohesion of life-minded souls, a community to lead us through the darkest of times.

My heritage is in the northern spiritual traditions, specifically druidry, shamanism, and alchemy.

I bring these into modernity through the agencies and disciplines of medicine, depth psychology, and magic.

My landscape is now Australia; working with people and culture to forge a new identity and direction; clarifying meaning and purpose; grounded in ritual and ceremony, and the offerings that unfold; a direction encapsulated in the beating heart.

Contact details: drkennan1@gmail.com

www.ingramcontent.com/pod-product-compliance
Lightning Source LLC
Chambersburg PA
CBHW030034100526
44590CB00011B/200